D0293060

ALSO BY GENIE JAMES, M.M.Sc.
& C. W. RANDOLPH, JR., M.D.

From Hormone Hell to Hormone Well

From Belly Fat to Belly Flat

GENIE JAMES, M.M.Sc.
AND C. W. RANDOLPH, Jr., M.D.

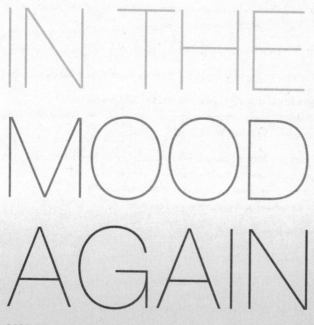

IN THE
MOOD
AGAIN

USE THE POWER OF HEALTHY HORMONES
TO REBOOT YOUR SEX LIFE—AT ANY AGE

A FIRESIDE BOOK
Published By Simon & Schuster
NEW YORK LONDON TORONTO SYDNEY

Fireside
A Division of Simon & Schuster, Inc.
1230 Avenue of the Americas
New York, NY 10020

Copyright © 2010 by Women Evolving LLC

All rights reserved, including the right to reproduce this book
or portions thereof in any form whatsoever. For information address
Fireside Subsidiary Rights Department, 1230 Avenue of the Americas,
New York, NY 10020

First Fireside paperback edition January 2010

Fireside and colophon are registered trademarks of Simon & Schuster, Inc.

For information about special discounts for bulk purchases,
please contact Simon & Schuster Special Sales at 1-866-506-1949
or business@simonandschuster.com.

The Simon & Schuster Speakers Bureau can bring authors to your live event.
For more information or to book an event contact the
Simon & Schuster Speakers Bureau at 1-866-248-3049
or visit our website at www.simonspeakers.com.

Designed by Ruth Lee-Mui

Manufactured in the United States of America

10 9 8 7 6 5 4 3 2 1

Library of Congress Cataloging-in-Publication Data
James, Genie.
    In the mood again / Genie James & C.W. Randolph.
      p.   cm.
    "A Fireside Book."
    1. Sexual desire disorders—Popular works.   2. Sex therapy—Popular
works.   3. Hormone therapy—Popular works.   4. Women—Health and
hygiene—Popular works.   I. Randolph, C.W.   II. Title.
    RC560.S46J36   2009
    615'.366—dc22   2009012077

ISBN 978-1-4391-4916-4
ISBN 978-1-4391-5567-7 (eBook)

NOTE TO READERS

This publication is based on the medical, professional, and clinical expertise of its authors and contains their opinions and ideas. It is sold with the understanding that the authors and publisher are not engaged in rendering medical, health, or any kind of professional services in this book. The information provided herein is for informational purposes only and is not intended as a substitute for advice from your physician or other health care professional. You should not use the information within these pages for diagnosis or treatment of any health problem or for prescription of any medication or other treatment. You should consult with a health care professional before starting any diet, exercise program, natural product supplementation, before taking any medication, or if you have or suspect you might have a health problem. You should not stop taking any medication without consulting your physician.

In addition, the authors sometimes recommend particular

websites and reference materials as information sources. All recommendations within the text were made independent of any affiliation. The authors also encourage readers to take responsibility for their personal health education and seek out other reference materials and websites offering a difference of opinion or approach to hormone health and sexual vitality.

The authors and publisher specifically disclaim all responsibility for any liability, loss or risk, personal or otherwise, which is incurred as a consequence, directly or indirectly, of the use and application of any of the contents of this book.

In memory of my grandmother, Nellie Floy Williams,
who in her 70s once told me:
"Honey, always try to look pretty when you go to bed and
never forget that there are a hundred and
one ways for a man and a woman to make love."

CONTENTS

INTRODUCTION

If your sex drive is in the toilet (and has been for longer than you care to admit) and the idea of a long night of steamy lovemaking seems as current as eight-track tapes, then this book is for you. More than likely, you enjoyed a robust sex life in your 20s, but as the years have gone by, you have increasingly felt too tired, too old, or simply not in the mood for sex. You have bought into the myth that as the decades stack up, less frequent and less pleasurable sex is a sad fact of life. Well, stay tuned, because we are here to present you with a new reality.

No matter how old you are or how long it has been since you felt in the mood, you can once again enjoy regular, passionate, and relationship-enriching sex. Even better, your renewed sex life can become a secret fountain of youth, giving you more energy, helping you lose weight, and improving your overall health and well-being.

Sound too good to be true? It's not. Worried that you will

need handfuls of expensive, side effect–ridden prescription drugs? You won't. Afraid that we are going to recommend you try getting turned on by porn or experiment with some form of gymnastic erotica? Don't be. Whether you are 30-something and suffering from double-income-no-sex (DINS) syndrome, 40-something and choosing to change channels rather than get frisky, 50-something and having too many hot flashes to even consider stirring up any action between the sheets, or 60-something and avoiding sex because of performance issues, your sex life can be better than ever before. Read on to find out how.

You Are Not Alone

If your sex life has been on pause, you have lots of company. The number of Americans leading low-sex/no-sex lives is startling. I (Genie James) first became aware of the scale of our nation's low-libido epidemic in 2002 when I collaborated with C. W. (Randy) Randolph, Jr., M.D., my coauthor and husband, to write *From Hormone Hell to Hormone Well.* Part of my research involved documenting the link between hormone imbalance and quality-of-life issues. Over a six-month period, I interviewed more than two hundred new male and female patients ranging in age from 30 to 70.

Most of the reported issues were expected: less energy, weight gain, hot flashes, saggy skin, foggy thinking, and/or depression. My lightning bolt was that sexual dysfunction—loss of sex drive or libido, performance problems, and/or decreased sexual pleasure—was the number one issue for 66 percent of respondents. Worse, resignation to an increasingly sexless life was a common theme. Here are some excerpts from my interviews:

I used to enjoy sex a lot. Even after marriage and a couple of kids, I could get in the mood at the drop of a hat. My husband and I had the habit of making love two to three times a week in the morning before we woke our children up. That was until I turned 35. I still love my husband, but now when he wakes me up at six o'clock in the morning, I just get annoyed.

—*Sharon, 39 years old*

I have been divorced for almost fourteen years now. For the first few years, I was a real Casanova. I particularly loved to take a woman I was dating on a cruise. My favorite thing was to have wild sex on our stateroom's balcony. Then, about four years ago, I began to have difficulty getting and keeping an erection. I became embarrassed. While I still ask women out for dinner and a movie, it has been two years since I had sex. Occasionally I masturbate, but even that doesn't give me much pleasure.

—*Edward, 55 years old*

Me want to have sex? You must be kidding. I am 27 pounds heavier than I was thirty years ago, my droopy bosoms hang down to my navel, and you could balance a six-pack on my rear end. The bottom line is that my husband and I haven't had sex in eleven years. He used to fool around outside our marriage, but with my body, I couldn't blame him. Lately, however, he, too, seems to have run out of gas. We spend most nights sitting on the sofa flipping channels and eating nachos. I guess that is some kind of intimacy, right?

—*Nadine, 61 years old*

A review of large-scale clinical studies indicated that I had tapped into a national trend. The statistics were daunting:

- Twenty million couples have stopped being sexually intimate.
- Forty million Americans live in a no-sex or low-sex marriage.
- 43 percent of women and 31 percent of men suffer sexual inadequacy due to low desire, performance anxiety, premature ejaculation, pain during intercourse, or other reasons.

Interestingly, these statistics may actually be underestimates of sexual dysfunction in the United States. Loss of libido was the second most common sexual dysfunction in men. The first was premature ejaculation. In another medical survey, doctors reported that about 50 percent of women from ages 28 to 60 say they no longer derive pleasure from sexual activities.

My goodness, I thought. America is in the midst of a low-sex/no-sex epidemic with no cure in sight. But believing that great sex is only a playground for the young-in-years is dead-wrong thinking. For decades, we have medically proven that you can turn back the clock and have an active and enjoyable sex life at any age. It is time we told the world.

The idea for this book was born.

Our Medically Proven Promise

If you want a better sex life, Randy and I are exceptionally qualified to help. No matter what your age or how long it has been since you initiated and/or enjoyed wonderful sex, we offer more than hope. We have two natural solutions that can either intersect or stand alone. Both approaches begin and end with your hormones.

Human sexuality is a complex biological phenomenon that is controlled at a cellular level by your body's hormones. The ovaries and testes are the body's factory for the three sex hormones: estrogen, progesterone, and testosterone. When all three sex hormones are produced in optimum amounts, you are easily aroused and sexual performance is a delight.

As the ovaries and testes age, however, they manufacture less hormones. Declining hormone levels not only compromise libido and impair sexual performance, they also contribute to a host of other physical, emotional, and mental issues. Some symptoms, such as abdominal weight gain, extreme fatigue, hot flashes, night sweats, mood swings, depression, bloating, foggy thinking, and headaches, are uncomfortable. Others, such as an increased risk of heart disease, dementia, and breast, uterine, and prostate cancers, can be life threatening. Whew! With all that going on, who would be in the mood?

Our good news: You don't have to resign yourself to getting fat, ornery, sick, and increasingly sexless. If you safely and naturally replenish deteriorating hormone levels, you can feel like your youthful self again. Not only will your sex life return with a bang, your body will be healthier with more muscle and less fat.

Our first approach to restoring your sex drive and improving your health involves replacing the hormones your body is missing with ones just like it used to make. Let us be clear: This is *not* accomplished by prescribing the popular synthetic hormones, such as Premarin or Prempro. In order to be patented, the molecular structure of these hormones has been altered to be slightly different from the ones produced within the body. Though slight, the difference can be deadly. The 2002 Women's Health Initiative (WHI) study linked synthetic hormones to an increased risk of breast and uterine cancers, heart attack, stroke, and Alzheimer's disease.

We use a different type of hormone—bioidentical hormone replacement therapy (BHRT)—to treat hormone deficiencies. *Bioidentical* refers to plant-derived hormone molecules that are identical to the human hormones produced within your body. Hormone receptors from the genitals to the brain recognize, receive, and utilize bioidentical hormones like a key fitting into and turning a lock.

Randy's expertise in BHRT is unique. Prior to attending medical school, he was a licensed compounding pharmacist with a deep interest in pharmacognosy, which is the study of medicine derived from natural sources such as plants and herbs. Long before the WHI study in 2002, he recognized the side effects triggered by synthetic hormones and chose BHRT as a safer and more effective alternative. For more than a decade, Randy has used BHRT to treat thousands of women and men suffering from low libido and/or sexual performance problems.

After only three months on an individualized prescription of BHRT, 92 percent of Randy's male and female patients report a complete restoration of sexual desire; 97 percent of women say they no longer have vaginal dryness and pain with intercourse; 88 percent of men report that erectile dysfunction is no longer an issue. As a testimony to BHRT's additional health benefits, 99 percent of all patients indicate they have more energy and 87 percent say they have lost 10 pounds or more.

In response to new medical evidence combined with a groundswell of consumer awareness and demand, BHRT has gained enormous popularity in the last decade. Still, if you are interested in pursuing BHRT as a treatment for low libido and other symptoms of hormone imbalance, you may face some challenges. You will first have to find a doctor who is trained and experienced in prescribing it. While more and more doctors are attending continuing medical education programs to learn about this emerging field of medicine, the number of BHRT specialists in the United States is not yet sufficient to meet an ever-increasing demand.

Cost can also be an issue. Our medical center accepts most health insurance plans, but many BHRT specialists serve only self-pay patients. The out-of-pocket cost can range from hundreds to thousands of dollars.

Some approaches to bioidentical hormone replacement are more controversial than others. For instance, some physicians prescribe dosages of bioidentical hormones that elevate levels above the physiologic, or normal, level, causing women in their 50s, 60s, and beyond to keep having periods. We do not advocate this approach. Also, it is important to make sure that the hormones are truly bioidentical. There are a number of cheaper counterfeits on the market today.

BHRT is a great option for restoring youthful sexual function, but it is not yet a panacea for all. If you are wondering whether hormone replacement is for you, we provide a checklist of factors to help you sort through your options. If your informed decision is to move forward, we give advice on how to find a medical professional in your area worthy of your trust.

Not sure if BHRT is for you? Don't give up on your sex life yet. Randy and I offer an alternative approach to boosting your lagging hormone levels.

For more than twenty years, I have been exploring natural approaches to women's health, consulting with hospitals and physicians across the country. My focus on female sexual desire, sexual function, and sexual response began more than fifteen years ago in response to the rapid increase in women's longevity. Recognizing that women could spend up to a third of their lives in a menopausal state, I knew it was time to move beyond traditional thinking to develop a natural and easily accessible approach to maintaining healthy levels of sexual desire and fulfillment for life. Over time, I developed an integrated approach that merged the fields of neurology, psychology, and nutrition.

When I first lobbied doctors about natural approaches to boosting lagging hormone levels, I faced stiff opposition. Then and now, most conventional physicians cling to the ideas that there is no such thing as too much estrogen in women and testosterone is a male-only hormone. Abundant scientific evidence in the United States and Europe has proven this thinking incorrect and dangerous.

Popular pharmaceutical treatments, such as antidepressants and synthetic hormones, mask the symptoms but don't resolve the underlying issue of declining hormone levels. Based on centuries-old wisdom and groundbreaking clinical studies, I developed an alternative approach to boosting hormone levels. This three-step program combines a hormone-healthy diet with clinically tested nutritional supplements and specific lifestyle choices. It is simple, accessible, and relatively inexpensive. Best of all, it works fabulously.

You'll see references in this book to many scientific studies that back up our recommendations. But Randy and I have our own focus group: Since 2003, we have tracked the response of more than seven hundred women and men. After two months, 97 percent of women committing to the three steps report significant improvements in sexual function, including desire, arousal, lubrication, satisfaction, and orgasm. An increase in desire before physical stimulation is reported by 94 percent of men. This is a particularly exciting statistic, since prescription erectile dysfunction (ED) drugs, such as Viagra and Cialis, stimulate blood flow to the penis but do nothing to restore arousal. In our focus group, 86 percent of men who previously took an ED prescription report that after only six weeks, their erections are consistently harder and longer lasting than ever before.

Hormone health and great sex don't need to be a confusing puzzle. This book makes it easy by giving you food and supplement suggestions, as well as lifestyle tips.

Better Sex, Healthier Body, Happier Relationships

Here's more good news: Restoring your body's optimum hormone balance, improving your libido, and having sex two to three times a week can do you a world of good in ways you might not have anticipated.

Medical studies show that restoring youthful hormone levels improves overall health, reduces the risk of heart disease and cancer, promotes weight loss and healthy body composition, and increases energy and vitality. Sexually active men and women in their 50s, 60s, and 70s report having more youthful-looking skin, shinier hair, and whiter teeth. Just as exciting, clinical studies have found that people who have sex two or more times a week live longer.

More sex has also been linked to enhanced intimacy. Men

who have more frequent sex say they feel closer to their partner and enjoy the nuances of intimacy, such as talking, cuddling, and foreplay, as much as the main event. Women who find themselves in the mood again are more willing to put down their to-do lists to play out sexual fantasies or experiment with new techniques or positions.

Here's to Your (Sexual) Health

In 2009, I turned 50 and Randy turned 60. I can honestly say that our relationship gets hotter with each passing year and we feel great. We want you to be able to say the same. I hope you find the answers you need in this book. To ask us questions or to tell us about your own experiences with this program, visit us at www.hormonewell.com.

Part One:

Why Have I Lost the Urge?

My guess is that you have opened this book because the title caught your eye. You used to enjoy a great sex life, but you've lost that sizzle between the sheets. Your lovemaking is increasingly infrequent, and on the rare occasion when you do have sex, it just isn't as much fun as it used to be. In fact, it hardly seems worth the trouble.

You blame your dwindling sex drive on age, stress, weight gain, and/or fatigue. You are almost resigned to a future of ho-hum hand holding and good-night pecks on the cheek, but every once in a while you think back to your sexually robust 20s and wonder *what happened*. Why have you lost the urge?

In Part One, you'll learn that love is not your answer and age alone is not your problem. Odds are that you have a medical condition that is sabotaging your sex life at a cellular level. Declining levels of the body's three sex hormones—estrogen, progesterone, and testosterone—are the primary reason your sex drive has gone down the tubes.

In Chapter 1, you'll see that women are the first to experience a shift in hormone production. As early as the mid-30s, a medical condition called estrogen dominance causes a drop in female libido and arousal. Then, in your 40s and 50s, a loss of testosterone can sap any remaining sexual energy. As you move into menopause, your body's inner estrogen seesaw dips down instead of up. Irregular or no periods is one sign of low estrogen levels; vaginal dryness and thinning of the vaginal walls are others. Wondering if your aging ovaries are the culprits silently sabotaging your sex life? Our ten-question quiz will help you find out. Chapter 1 concludes with a description of how age-related hormone imbalance is much more than a sexual nuisance; if undiagnosed and untreated, it can significantly increase the risk of female cancers, heart disease, and Alzheimer's.

Chapter 2 puts male hormone production under the microscope. You'll learn the medical reason that former between-the-sheets enthusiasts start to lose interest after 40. Even more important, you'll be enlightened (and probably frightened) by research linking declining testosterone levels to erectile dysfunction, prostate cancer, and cardiovascular disease.

While an age-related decline in hormone levels is the most common cause of low libido, your sex drive could be the victim of other silent culprits. Chapter 3 describes how stress, weight gain, sleeplessness, and environmental toxins can upset your body's optimum hormone balance and squelch desire. Already wondering whether your stressful, sleepless life is the reason you've lost both your hormones and that desire? Chapter 3 concludes with questions to help you evaluate your lifestyle.

1

Ladies First

As soon as Randy and I signed our publishing contract, I called my sister Sheila to share the good news.

"You're writing a book about sex?" she asked in the same horrified voice she used when she first learned I took all my clothes off before a massage. "You can't do that. We weren't raised to talk about those things. Mother would roll over in her grave. You will just have to tear that book contract up."

I knew I had set myself up. For fifty-odd years, my sister and I had been playing out different versions of the same script.

"Sheila," I responded, "this book has a very important message. Healthy sexual function is an essential component of a quality life, helping to promote positive body image and maintain strong intimate connections with partners. Unfortunately, most women have the misconception that great sex is a playground for only the young-in-years. The medical reality is women can enjoy regular and pleasurable sex through their 50s, 60s, 70s, and even beyond."

"Genie," she said with a sigh, "there are television commercials galore about drugs that help men with their penis problems. When it comes to women, however, it's not that simple. We need desire, energy, as well as the willingness to unclothe a body with some road miles on it. And what if all our private parts don't work like they used to? What fun is that? Unless you are writing this book for young women in their 20s, you won't have any readers. When a woman gets past a certain age, she is just *not in the mood*."

"Sheila," I replied, "that is *exactly* the point."

The "Curse" Through the "Change"

For centuries, a woman's menstrual cycle has been regarded as a blessing and a curse. The onset of menstruation signals the beginning of the reproductive years. In biblical times, menstruating women were regarded as unclean and were housed separately from their families for the duration of their period. In contrast, pregnant women were coddled and celebrated. Their missed periods signaled new life and perpetuation of the clan. When menstruation ceased once and for all, however, women were again ostracized because their greatest use—reproduction—was over. From menopause until death, their womanhood was usurped as they were considered dried-up old crones.

Contemporary women have long since proven that their worth is defined by much more than their body's ability to serve as a baby factory. We are also the beneficiaries of the 1960s sexual revolution spurred by the launch of the Pill. Readily available contraception set us free to claim and enjoy our bodies as sexual instruments designed for pleasure as well as reproduction. And increased longevity is giving us many more years to have fun in the sack. So, what has gone wrong? Why doesn't sex get better with age?

If your once great sex life has become only a fond memory, stop feeling guilty and don't give up. Your decreased sex drive is likely linked to your periods, or lack of. The same hormones that stimulated you to menstruate and begin your transformation from child to woman as they surged in puberty are now causing your libido to plummet as they recede in midlife.

Hormones are chemicals within your body that transfer information and instructions from one cell to another. Often described as the body's chemical messengers, hormones travel through the bloodstream to hormone receptor sites throughout the body, including the brain.

The ovaries and testes produce three sex hormones: estrogen, progesterone, and testosterone. Biochemically, the cholesterol molecule is the building block for all three sex hormones. These hormones work together to stimulate growth and development, support reproduction, regulate metabolism, and fuel your sex drive. A surge of hormones first caused us to mature into adults capable of reproduction. We then age because levels of these same hormones decline.

When young, healthy ovaries produce optimum amounts of all three sex hormones, the body is said to be in hormonal equilibrium, or balance. A woman with balanced hormones feels sexy, energetic, and optimistic. Her body is fit, toned, easily lubricated, and frequently aroused. Her hair is shiny and her teeth sparkle brightly when she smiles. She smiles a lot because she has frequent and multiple orgasms. Don't hate this woman. She is you in your 20s.

Puberty Through the Early Reproductive Years

Puberty is the time of life when hormones stimulate growth and maturation needed for reproduction. For girls, this begins with their first period. In the United States, the average age of first menstrual bleeding, or period, is 11.75 years.[1]

The onset of puberty initiates a chain reaction of hormone activity. The body releases a hormone called gonadotropin-releasing hormone (GnRH). When GnRH reaches the pituitary gland (a pea-shaped gland that sits just under the brain), this gland releases two more hormones: luteinizing hormone (LH) and follicle-stimulating hormone (FSH). LH and FSH stimulate the ovaries to begin producing all three sex hormones, but estrogen has the greatest influence. *Estrogen* is actually an umbrella term for three different types of estrogen produced by the ovaries: estriol (E3), which accounts for 60 to 80 percent of circulating estrogen; estradiol (E2), which accounts for 10 to 20 percent of circulating estrogen; and estrone (E1), which accounts for 3 to 5 percent of circulating estrogen.

Gradually increasing estrogen levels cause girls to grow into women. The lower half of the pelvis, including the hips, widens to form a birth canal. Other physical changes caused by estrogen include breast development and more fatty tissue distributed on the hips, buttocks, thighs, upper arms, and pubis. Pubic hair begins to grow and vaginal walls become thicker and pinker. In a monthly menstrual cycle, two things happen: (1) Estrogen levels rise slowly during the first half of the month, spike right before ovulation (around day fourteen), and then gradually fall off again just before the period; (2) progesterone levels rise sharply after ovulation and then fall off just before the period.

From puberty, progesterone functions to maintain the uterus and prepare it for pregnancy. If an ovum, or egg, is fertilized, progesterone is also produced by the placenta to help change the lining of the uterus so that the interior cells will provide nutrition to the developing embryo. If conception fails to occur, the drop in progesterone and estrogen levels in the blood leads to a shedding of the lining of the uterus, or a period.

Progesterone not only supports a healthy pregnancy, it is also the hormone most associated with a positive quality of life. It is frequently called the feel-good hormone because of its calming and positive effect on moods and feelings of well-being. Progesterone's relaxing effect helps you to sleep better. It also acts as a natural diuretic. This hormone plays the critical role of balancing or neutralizing estrogen's propensity to promote cell growth, which if left unchecked can be a precursor to cancer. Many studies validate how optimum progesterone levels can have a cancer-protective effect. In addition, progesterone stimulates bone growth.

Most women are aware of how the dynamic dance between estrogen and progesterone shifts as they age, but they tend to think of testosterone as a male-only hormone. It is not. From puberty until menopause, the female body produces on average one-tenth of the amount of testosterone produced by the male body. Testosterone in females contributes to the rapid growth spurt at puberty and is believed to help regulate the function of the reproductive tract, kidneys, liver, and muscles. When it comes to sexual growth and function, testosterone is best known as the hormone of desire. In addition to fueling libido, it promotes sexual pleasure by causing the nipples and clitoris to be sensitive to touch.

Your Three Sex Hormones: From Puberty to Age 30

Estrogen	Progesterone	Testosterone
Source: Ovaries and body fat	Source: Ovaries, adrenal glands, and placenta when pregnant	Source: Ovaries and adrenal glands
• Develops the sex organs and secondary sex characteristics such as breasts and pubic hair • Maintains the menstrual cycle • Supports the growth and function of the uterus, specifically creating the lining of the uterus to prepare it for pregnancy • Stimulates cell growth	• Maintains the uterus and prepares it for pregnancy • Promotes survival of the egg once it is fertilized • Stimulates bone building • Acts as a normal diuretic • Serves as a natural antidepressant • Promotes regular sleep patterns • Opposes estrogen's predisposition to promote cell growth, which if left unchecked can be a precursor to cancer • Helps maintain libido	• Boosts libido • Increases energy • Maintains muscle mass and healthy body composition • Strengthens bones • Causes the nipples and clitoris to be sensitive to touch and sexual pleasure

The Reproductive Years

The early reproductive stage begins with a girl's first period and lasts until she is in her early 30s. For the most part, if periods occur on a normal twenty-eight-day cycle, it can be inferred that the ovaries are producing plenty of all three sex hormones. Some young women may experience premenstrual syndrome, or PMS, although it is more likely to occur once a woman is in her 30s. Bloating, anxiety, irritability, back pain, nausea, cramping, and lethargy are some of the most common PMS symptoms.

Biologically, the human species is wired to reproduce. Many women in their reproductive years say their periods affect their sex drive in unexpected ways. Research shows that women tend to feel lustier and flirtier, fantasize more about sex, and initiate sex more during ovulation. Surveys of women under 30 found that 94 percent reported feeling more attractive during the time of month they were most fertile.[2]

If you loved having lots of steamy sex in your youth, balanced hormones were the reason. Whether or not you had babies in mind, your sex hormones were clamoring for you to get pregnant.

Premenopause

Natalie, a 42-year-old mother of three, came to our Ageless and Wellness Center because she missed having great sex. She complained of low libido and difficulty reaching orgasm:

> I was 34 when Dan and I had our third child. We felt our family was complete, so he decided to have a vasectomy. Not having to worry about birth control helped me enjoy sex more than ever before. Dan was delighted that for the first time in our relationship, I was initiating sex several times a week. I always enjoyed multiple orgasms. Dan used to call me the "doing-it diva."
>
> Since turning 40, however, things have changed. I have absolutely no interest in or energy for sex. In the evenings, I tell Dan I am too tired, and in the mornings I get mad if he won't leave me alone and let me sleep. On the rare occasions when we do have sex, I don't climax. Dan wants us to go to a marriage counselor, but I think something might be medically wrong with me. That's why I came here. Can you tell me what is really going on?

Natalie was right to think she was suffering from a medical condition. Her sex life was being sabotaged by her aging ovaries.

Premenopause is the beginning of a gradual slowing down of the reproductive cycle. Typically this occurs in the mid-30s through the mid- to late 40s. Young women having regular periods are frequently unaware that their ovaries' production of much-needed hormones has begun to shift. Consider Brenda, a 37-year-old mother of two, who contacted me through our Web site:

> Ms. James, a friend forwarded me your newsletter describing how low hormone levels can cause a woman to lose her sex drive. I still have a period every month, so my body is obviously still making enough hormones. Still, something is going on, because I used to crave lots of sex and now I cringe at the thought.
>
> When my husband and I met eleven years ago, we would spend entire weekends either loving it up in bed or running around the house naked. For the past three or four years, however, it has been increasingly hard for me to get turned on, even though my husband seems always ready to go. I put him off as long as possible. When we do have sex, I feel about as much excitement as when I fold clothes. I expected this at menopause but not now. I'm too young for my sex drive to have completely dried up, aren't I?

Many women like Brenda in their early to mid-30s think they are too young to be suffering from imbalanced hormone levels. But, in fact, Brenda's hormone decline and loss of sex drive was right on time.

The biological fact is that female hormone levels begin to decline ten to fifteen years before the onset of menopause. From the mid-30s until the late 40s, the ovaries continue to produce sufficient estrogen for regular periods, but they produce less and less progesterone. In fact, progesterone levels fall 120 times more rapidly than estrogen levels.

Estrogen dominance is the clinical term for this condition of relatively high estrogen levels compared to increasingly low progesterone levels. For the premenopausal woman, loss of libido is one of the first symptoms of estrogen dominance. Fatigue, moodiness, worsened PMS, headaches, memory fog, and abdominal weight gain are others.

Although their ovaries and adrenal glands are still pumping out lots of testosterone, premenopausal women can also suffer from a condition of relative testosterone deficiency. This occurs because levels of another hormone, called sexual hormone-binding globulin (SHBG), increase two to three times normal levels. SHBG then binds to free testosterone molecules circulating within the body and, in doing so, keeps the testosterone from fulfilling its mission of fueling sex drive at a cellular level.

Premenopausal women complaining of decreased sex drive are frequently misdirected and misdiagnosed. Male partners might suggest new lingerie or a night on the town. Commiserating friends might advise that the problem is age related and will only get worse. Most doctors, if they listen at all, offer patronizing advice or a prescription for an antidepressant or sleeping pill. The end result: more frustration and guilt but no more sex.

Perimenopause

Perimenopause literally means the time "around menopause" that occurs between the mid- to late 40s and early 50s. These are the years when the ovaries' production of estrogen begins to sputter. Fluctuating estrogen levels cause periods to be irregular. Some women will menstruate for three full weeks, whereas others will go two to four months without a period. This transition stage can last from two to eight years. If you are in perimeno-pause, you could be estrogen dominant or estrogen deficient.

Though estrogen levels begin to decline, that does not mean all perimenopausal women immediately become estrogen defi-cient. Remember that estrogen dominance is a relative condition of too much estrogen with too little progesterone. Some peri-menopausal women's estrogen levels decline so slowly that their estrogen-to-progesterone ratio still qualifies them as estrogen dominant. Other perimenopausal women continue to be estro-gen dominant because extra body fat is continuing to produce lots of estrogen even when their ovaries can't.

In Chapter 5, I will discuss how specific hormone-measuring laboratory tests definitely resolve whether you are estrogen dominant or deficient. Without testing, your vagina is a good barometer. Estrogen deficiency causes vaginal dryness and thinning of the vaginal wall. If you are having difficulty lubri-cating before and during sex or if intercourse has become painful, your vagina is letting you know that it is lacking much-needed estrogen.

These are the years when your ovaries' production of testos-terone also begins to decline. Testosterone deficiency (also medi-cally termed androgen insufficiency) catalyzes a shift from low libido to no libido. If you add together an extra 20 or 30 pounds, hot flashes, night sweats, insomnia, vaginal dryness, and a fre-quent need to pee, it is quickly understandable why many peri-menopausal women prefer flipping channels to fondling between the sheets.

Menopause

In years past, sexuality after menopause notoriously received little attention from the traditional medical community. Many women hesitated to report low libido or problems with arousal or sensation because they were embarrassed or doubted that their doctors would have the time or interest to address it. Today, 42 million postmenopausal women in the United States realize they might live another 30 to 40 years. They want to know: "Why should I go without sex for one-third of my life?" They are demanding that libido and sexual function be a central component in their medical strategy for healthy aging. The problem is that many physicians don't know how to reverse the negative impact that hormone level decline has on libido and other aspects of female sexual health.

You are not officially menopausal until you have not had a period for at least twelve months. The average age of American women entering natural menopause is 51. Menopause, or "the change," marks the end of fertility. The pituitary glands and the hypothalamus continue to produce their hormones (GnRH, FSH, and LH), but the ovaries are no longer able to produce enough estrogen to ovulate.

Too often, traditional medical professionals treat menopause as an age-related disease, like high blood pressure or Alzheimer's. Menopause is not a disease; it is a stage of life. Many doctors also have the misconception that once a woman enters menopause, her ovaries turn off like a light switch, causing all hormone production to cease. This is not true. Progesterone production continues to decline, but the ovaries of some menopausal women continue to produce between 40 and 60 percent of the estrogen and testosterone produced by premenopausal women.

Once again, hormone balance is relative. If the ovaries' production of testosterone does not slow down in tandem with estrogen and progesterone levels, women become comparatively testosterone dominant. When testosterone production continues to outstrip estrogen and progesterone production, women may get whiskers, male pattern baldness, and a chronically low voice.

As levels of all three sex hormones dip lower, some menopausal women report more severe symptoms of sexual dysfunction, such as a phobic aversion to sexual contact with a chosen sexual partner or involuntary spasm of the outer area of the vagina, interfering with vaginal penetration. These sexual disorders are frequently misdiagnosed. Heather, who is 53 years old, explained her situation:

> These should be the happiest, most relaxed years of our lives, but my problems with sex are making me and my husband miserable. Before menopause, we enjoyed rambunctious sex at least two times a week. Now, instead of getting excited about an upcoming bedroom adventure, I dread feeling my husband's hand on my skin. Worse, the minute he reaches for me, my vagina snaps shut as if on a spring lock.
>
> My doctor says there is nothing physically wrong with me. She diagnosed me as suffering from empty nest syndrome and recommended I take up a new hobby. My husband has tried to be understanding, but his patience is wearing thin. If I don't figure this out soon, I am afraid of what might happen to our marriage.

Regardless of whether a menopausal woman experiences slightly uncomfortable physical symptoms—like hot flashes or night sweats—or more extreme symptoms—such as those experienced by Heather—hormone imbalance is the culprit. Sexual desire, pleasure, and performance will only be restored once the equilibrium among all sex hormones—estrogen, progesterone, *and testosterone*—is restored.

Hysterectomy: The Sudden Shock of Artificial Menopause

Hysterectomy is the second most common major surgery performed on women in the United States. (The most common is cesarean section delivery.) Most hysterectomies are performed on women between the ages of 30 and 49. Each year, more than six hundred thousand women experience the sudden shock of entering artificial menopause as a result of a partial or total hysterectomy.[3]

In a partial hysterectomy, only the uterus is removed, and the ovaries are left in place. However, because of reduced blood circulation to the ovaries, production of the sex hormones is compromised. In a total hysterectomy, the uterus, fallopian tubes, and ovaries are removed, which results in the cessation of all ovarian hormone production. Small amounts of estrogen and testosterone will continue to be produced by body fat and the adrenal glands.

There are several reasons women are advised to consider an elective hysterectomy. The most common are heavy bleeding, large fibroids, endometrial polyps, endometriosis, and other endometrium issues. Some women just want a hysterectomy for comfort (to eliminate the discomfort associated with PMS, menstrual cramping, or irregular bleeding) or for a prolapsed uterus (a condition in which the pelvic organs drop). More dire indications include cancers of the uterus or ovaries—conditions that truly merit immediate surgery.

Too many physicians make the mistake of prescribing only

estrogen for women after a hysterectomy, but estrogen alone is not enough. After a hysterectomy, a woman's body lacks its primary factory of all three sex hormones.

An Important Note About DHEA

This chapter has addressed how an age-related decline in sex hormones negatively impacts your libido and feelings of arousal and sexual pleasure. Dehydroepiandrosterone (DHEA) is another hormone that influences the levels of your sex hormones, thereby also influencing your sex drive.

The adrenal glands produce the majority of DHEA while the ovaries contribute a minimal amount of this powerful steroid hormone. It is the most abundant steroid hormone in the body. DHEA is called a precursor hormone because it can be converted to testosterone. Levels of DHEA naturally decrease with age. By the time you are 80 years old, your DHEA levels will be about 5 to 10 percent of the amount produced during your reproductive years. Age is not the only factor influencing DHEA production. Chapter 3 will explain how chronic stress also depletes DHEA levels.

Surveys have linked declining DHEA production in women with a decreasing tendency to think about or initiate sex, as well as a decrease in feelings of sexual satisfaction.

Hormone Imbalance Affects Your Sex Life

From the mid-30s on, hormone imbalance can shove you into a virtual sexual quicksand. Your lack of sex drive is one big problem, but as additional symptoms stack up, your sex life is increas-

Symptoms of Hormone Imbalance			
Symptoms of Estrogen Dominance Typically begins in a ♀'s early to mid-30s and continues into perimenopause (late 40s to early 50s); however, overweight ♀ can continue to be estrogen dominant through and after menopause.		**Symptoms of Testosterone Deficiency** Can begin in a ♀'s 30s as a result of ↑SHBG that can "lock up" circulating testosterone, but more typically occurs during perimenopause (late 40s to early 50s).	
SEXUAL	OTHER	SEXUAL	OTHER
• Low libido	• Fatigue • Weight gain • Worsened PMS • Bloating • Headaches • Moodiness • Depression • Fibrocystic breasts • Night sweats • Increased risk of breast cancer • Increased risk of uterine cancer	• Low libido • Hot flashes	• Loss of energy • Loss of muscle mass • Decreased arousal
Symptoms of Estrogen Deficiency Typically occurs during the peri- and menopausal years.		**Symptoms of Testosterone Dominance** Typically occurs after menopause; the ovaries' production of testosterone remains relatively higher than declining estrogen and progesterone levels.	

(continued)

SEXUAL	OTHER	SEXUAL	OTHER

• Vaginal dryness
• Thinning of the
  vaginal wall
• Painful
  intercourse
	• Irregular
	  periods until
	  no more
	  periods at
	  all
			• Facial hair
			• Low voice
			• Male pattern
			  baldness

Declining DHEA Levels
Typically begins in a ♀'s early to mid-30s.

SEXUAL	
• Low libido • Less interest in initiating sex • Fewer sexual fantasies	

ingly compromised by a myriad of other interconnected physical, emotional, and mental issues. See the Symptoms of Hormone Imbalance table on page 17.

Answer the following questions to find out whether an age-related hormone imbalance could be killing your sex drive. If you answer yes to questions 1 and 2, or to at least three of the other questions, the odds are that your ovaries can no longer produce optimum levels of estrogen, progesterone, and testosterone.

1. Are you over 35 years of age?
2. Have you experienced a decrease in libido that has persisted for more than three months?
3. When your partner attempts to initiate sex, is boredom or dread more prominent than feelings of arousal?
4. Have you experienced two or more of the following symptoms of estrogen dominance for more than three months?

Weight gain	Hot flashes
Night sweats	Worsened PMS
Bloating	Headaches or migraines
Irregular bleeding	Fibrocystic breasts
Low energy/chronic fatigue	Sleep disturbance
Moodiness or depression	Memory loss or foggy thinking
Decrease in overall enjoyment of life	

5. Have your nipples or clitoris become less sensitive to stimulation?
6. Are you having problems with vaginal dryness?
7. Is intercourse painful?
8. Are you having difficulty climaxing even with manual or oral stimulation?
9. Are you officially menopausal (you have not had a period for more than one year) or have you had a partial or complete hysterectomy?
10. Has your voice changed to a lower timber or have you grown facial hair or begun to lose hair at the temples or crown?

Hormone Imbalance Puts Your Health at Risk

If the balance among your sex hormones has shifted, your sex life is not the only thing at risk. Your health is, too. Medical research has linked hormone imbalance to chronic health concerns, including cancer, heart disease, and Alzheimer's.

As previously described, one of estrogen's functions within the body is to foster cell proliferation or growth. Progesterone, however, inhibits cell growth. When progesterone levels begin to decline and the body becomes estrogen dominant, cell growth continues unchecked. Medical research has established estrogen dominance–stimulated cell growth as the underlying causative factor for endometriosis, PMS, polycystic ovary syndrome (PCOS), fibroids, fibrocystic breasts, as well as breast and uterine cancers. Because the word *cancer* strikes a chord of terror for most women, I want to discuss the relationship between estrogen dominance and cancer in greater detail.

Multiple studies show that women who develop breast cancer tend to have higher estrogen levels than women without breast cancer. Other studies have documented that women who were treated for breast cancer and continued to have high estrogen levels had a return of the disease sooner than breast cancer survivors with lower estrogen levels.[4]

One study found that women who start menstruating at an early age, or who enter menopause at a later age, are at greater risk for developing breast cancer. This data supports the theory that the number of menstrual cycles a woman has, and hence the length of exposure to estrogen during her lifetime, is a critical factor impacting breast cancer risk.[5]

Estrogen dominance can lead to breast cancer in one of two ways. The first has to do with the concentration of each of the three different forms of estrogen—estrone (E1), estradiol (E2), and estriol (E3)—circulating within the body. E1 and E2 both work within the body to increase expression of a gene (BCL-2) that causes cell division (development and growth), particularly in hormone-sensitive tissue such as the breast or uterine lining. If unchecked, this cell proliferation can lead to cancer. In fact, nearly every risk factor for breast and uterine cancers can be either directly or indirectly linked to an increase in E1, E2, or their receptor activity. A study published in the March 2008 issue of *Cancer Epidemiology, Biomarkers & Prevention* determined that high levels of E2 were associated with a significantly higher incidence of breast cancer recurrence.[6]

The second way that too much estrogen becomes a precursor for cancer has to do with how it is metabolized within the body. Researchers at Rockefeller University have found that the body metabolizes estrogen into several different metabolites, or estrogenic building blocks, which can impact cancer development.[7] Two metabolites, 2-hydroxyestrone and 2-hydroxyestradiol, tend to inhibit cancer growth. Another, 16-alpha-hydroxyestrone, actually encourages tumor development. Estrogen metabolism is determined by an individual's biochemical makeup, with some women producing more 2-hydroxy derivatives and others producing more 16-alpha-hydroxyestrone. Studies have shown that measuring the ratio of these two metabolites provides an important indication of risk for future development of estrogen-sensitive cancers.[8]

A variety of evidence suggests a link between estrogen dominance and migraine headaches, anxiety disorders, insomnia, and decreased mental acuity. Recent research has also suggested that an imbalance between estrogen and progesterone levels may be a precursor to Alzheimer's disease.

Testosterone deficiency can be another health concern for women. New medical evidence has identified testosterone deficiency as a key predictive factor for heart disease in women who

No, you are not losing your mind: you're just losing much-needed progesterone. When you don't have enough progesterone circulating, estrogen is the dominant hormone. Estrogen in overabundance makes you angry, edgy, short-tempered, and anxious. At the same time, estrogen increases the water content of the cells in your brain, making you groggy, fuzzy, and unfocused.

—Erika Schwartz, *The Hormone Solution*

have had hysterectomies.[9] Because heart disease is the leading cause of death for postmenopausal women, the time of life most associated with testosterone deficiency, researchers are continuing to explore how low testosterone levels contribute to a buildup of fatty material in the carotid artery.[10]

Hold on. Don't throw up your hands in despair, believing that your aging ovaries are dooming you to desire less and less sex as you get older. An age-related decline in the production of your sex hormones may be inevitable, but it is also reversible. Read on!

2

Mister, You Are Next

Thomas, a 44-year-old advertising executive and father of four, came to see Randy at the urging of his wife:

Dr. Randolph, I am embarrassed to admit that Samantha and I have only had sex three times in nine months. I love my wife very much and she is as beautiful as ever, but I simply have no interest. I can get an erection with physical stimulation, but it's not very firm and rarely lasts long enough for me to complete the deed. This is a big change for us. Up until two years ago, we had sex almost every morning.

I went to see my urologist, but he focused only on my erections, not my libido. He explained how one of the popular erectile dysfunction medications [such as Viagra, Cialis, or Levitra] could increase my body's production of nitric oxide, the chemical that causes blood vessels in the penis to relax, open, and produce an erection. I am not against taking a pill to give my penis some extra juice, but what about my other problem? What good is a hard-on if mentally I would rather be mowing the lawn than having sex? My wife thinks I might be going through some kind of male menopause. Does such a thing even exist?

Even though the concept is just starting to be understood, men also experience hormonal changes as they enter midlife. The medical term for this condition is *andropause*. It is a physiologic condition caused by an age-related decline in the male hormones, specifically testosterone from the testes, human growth hormone (HGH) from the pituitary, and dehydroepiandrosterone (DHEA) from the adrenal glands. When the male body is deficient in these hormones, sex doesn't seem as enticing and the physical act itself will not be up to par.

Thomas's urologist was ready to treat the symptom (erectile dysfunction) without addressing the underlying issue (decreased libido), which is an all-too-common phenomenon. Unfortunately, the conventional medical community has been slow to recognize the consequences of declining hormone levels in aging men.

The Truth About Male Menopause

The term *male menopause* has created controversy within the medical community. Menopause, by definition, means the end of menses. Ovulation ceases and female hormone production plummets over a relatively short time frame. In men, there is a more gradual decline in the production of male hormones, causing more subtle symptoms of varying severity. An androgen is defined as any steroid hormone that increases male characteristics.

Throughout this book, I use the term *andropause* because I feel it most adequately connotes a medical condition resulting from decreased androgen production.

Some physicians refer to this condition as *hypogonadism*, which does mean low hormone production, but young men can suffer from hypogonadism as well as older men. Other medical scientists refer to this condition as testosterone deficiency, androgen decline in the aging male (ADAM), or late-onset hypogonadism (LOH). Whatever the name, there is no denying the fact that andropause is a contemporary epidemic. According to the U.S. Census Bureau, approximately 13 million men currently suffer from symptoms of low testosterone.[1]

Your Youth: Rock Hard and Ready to Go

Like Thomas, your sex drive may have shifted from high gear to neutral or low. You may also have trouble getting and/or keeping an erection. If you are a man over 40, your sexual concerns are most likely caused by dipping testosterone levels. Testosterone is the sex hormone that men need not only to get in the mood but also to finish the act with a flourish rather than a fizzle.

Hormone production transforms little boys into young men. During male puberty, the hypothalamus secretes hormones that stimulate the pituitary gland to release hormones, which consist of follicle-stimulating hormone (FSH) and luteinizing hormone (LH). FSH stimulates development of the tubes in the testes in which sperm production takes place and is thought to be involved in sperm maturation. LH stimulates the testes to release testosterone.

Testosterone is the hormone primarily responsible for the

growth of the male sex organs, or genitals, including the penis, the duct system for sperm production and transport, and the accessory glands of the prostate and seminal vesicles. The first physical change occurs in the sex organs when the testes and scrotum begin to grow. The scrotum darkens, thickens, and drops to become pendulous. Approximately a year after testicular changes begin, the penis grows. It becomes longer and wider, taking years to reach its full size. Other hormone-driven changes include lengthening of the vocal cords, which causes the voice to deepen, and growth of pubic hair. Facial hair begins to appear on the face, chest, and abdomen.[2]

During puberty, most boys begin to experience sexual feelings and sensations. Sporadic and involuntary erections and wet dreams signal surging hormone levels. An increase in testosterone levels is also associated with an inclination to masturbate. To release the sexual tension associated with rising testosterone levels, nearly all boys masturbate at some point in their adolescence, some more frequently than others.

Testosterone levels peak in the 20s. During these years, most young men take hard, long-lasting erections for granted, and some report enjoying up to six or eight orgasms a day. Sexual fantasies abound, and when a partner is not available, masturbation is a ready second. Unfortunately, testosterone levels begin a slow downhill slide as early as age 30, dropping 1 percent a year on average. By the early 40s, testosterone deficiency can compromise both desire and performance. Levels decline even more rapidly after 50. An 80-year-old man will typically have only 20 to 50 percent of the level of testosterone he had at his peak. As the years go by, this gradual decline in testosterone is the biochemical reason that former between-the-sheets enthusiasts shift from enjoying sex several times a week to going through the motions a few times a year.

Not only is testosterone vital for sustaining proper erectile function and libido, it is also involved in building muscle, burning fat, maintaining energy, elevating mood, and maintaining bone density. Testosterone deficiency can lead to weight gain or obesity, loss of stamina and lean muscle mass, depression and anxiety, and an increased risk of diabetes and heart disease. Because a man's drop in testosterone is so gradual, the symptoms of andropause are frequently ignored or attributed to getting older.

Testosterone Deficiency Impacts Health and Mortality

Preston, a 54-year-old investment banker, was interested in scheduling a hormone consultation but had a few questions:

> I recently had lunch with a college friend I hadn't seen in twenty-five years. He was slim and full of energy. His new wife was a beautiful woman who looked to be in her early 30s. When I congratulated them on their marriage, she confided that they are trying to get pregnant. When she went to the restroom, I asked my old friend his secret. He said he started testosterone injections ten years ago and suggested I give it a try. I would like to get rid of my paunch, but I am concerned about the health risks. Isn't testosterone dangerous?

Preston is not alone in his concern. But the good news is that research backs up the claim that maintaining relatively high levels of testosterone can not only help men with their weight and libido, it can also contribute to leading a longer and healthier life.

Multiple medical studies have linked low testosterone levels with a higher death rate among men aged 50 or older. One study conducted at the University of Cambridge followed nearly twelve thousand men ranging in age from 40 to 79. After ten years, more than eight hundred of the men had died. After adjusting for factors that might increase risk of death—including age, weight, smoking, alcohol use, high blood pressure, diabetes, and physical activity—the link between low testosterone and earlier death remained. Compared to men with testosterone levels in the lowest quartile (25 percent), men in the highest quartile were 41 percent less likely to die.[3]

Similarly, a study conducted by medical researchers at the University of California–San Diego followed eight hundred men (ranging in age from 50 to 91 years old) from 1984 until death or 2004, whichever came first. Men with low testosterone levels were 33 percent more likely to die.

Cardiovascular Disease, Metabolic Syndrome, and Diabetes

Many studies have shown an association between low testosterone levels and a higher prevalence of heart disease. Lower testosterone levels are also associated with reduced pumping ability of the heart.

Growing research suggests that low testosterone levels may be intimately linked with insulin resistance and its related conditions of metabolic syndrome and diabetes.[4] Metabolic syndrome is a group of risk factors—high blood pressure, high blood sugar, unhealthy cholesterol levels, and abdominal fat—that make heart disease and diabetes more likely.[5]

Recent findings from the Third National Health and Nutrition Survey (NHANES III) demonstrated that men in the group with the lowest testosterone levels were approximately four times more likely to develop diabetes.

Prostate Cancer

June, a 54-year-old friend from our book club, lamented one evening:

> Genie, it's been two and a half years since Brad and I had sex. I really miss feeling close in that way. We used to have the most intimate conversations, um, you know . . . after. When our sex life first began to taper off, I would complain, but I stopped after Brad said to me: "Would you rather have sex or me die of prostate cancer?" His internist told him that his low sex drive was a signal that his body is making less testosterone, and while having less sex might be depressing, lower testosterone levels mean a lower risk of prostate cancer. Is that true?

I explained to June that Brad's internist is right about the link between his declining testosterone levels and his dwindled sex drive, but he's dead wrong in saying that low testosterone levels decrease a man's risk of prostate cancer. I put together some powerful medical research for her to share with her husband's doctor.

Each year, more than 186,000 American men learn they have prostate cancer. While most conventional physicians understand the link between declining testosterone production and decreased sex drive in men, many doctors—like Brad's internist—remain confused, thinking that low testosterone levels mean a decreased risk of prostate cancer and high testosterone levels are linked to an increased risk. Recent medical studies prove exactly the opposite.

In 2004, Abraham Morgentaler published a review in the *New England Journal of Medicine* validating that there was not a single study in human patients to suggest that raising testosterone levels increased the risk of prostate cancer.[6] This review challenged previously set thinking not only because the *New England Journal of Medicine* is one of the most prestigious medical journals, but also because Dr. Morgentaler's credentials as an associate clinical professor of urology at Harvard Medical School are highly respected.

Dr. Morgentaler's premise was further validated in 2008 by an article published in the *Journal of the National Cancer Institute*. Authors of eighteen separate studies from around the world pooled their data regarding the likelihood of developing prostate cancer based on concentrations of various hormones, including testosterone. This enormous study included more than three thousand men with prostate cancer and more than six thousand men without prostate cancer who served as controls in the study. No relationship was found between prostate cancer and any of the hormones studied, including total testosterone, free testosterone, and other minor androgens.[7]

In his groundbreaking book *Testosterone for Life*, Dr. Morgentaler states:

> New medical evidence indicates that men are actually at an increased risk of prostate cancer when they are older and their T [testosterone] levels have declined. Men never develop prostate cancer when they are young and their T levels are at their lifelong peak. New evidence suggests that low T, rather than high T, may be a risk for prostate cancer.[8]

Body, Mind, and Emotions

Rick, a 47-year-old retired tennis pro turned sportscaster, sat dejectedly looking at the floor during our conversation:

> I am here because I can't get it up anymore. I can't seem to get myself up, either. I used to run four to five miles every morning, but now I drag myself out of bed at the last minute, force myself to get dressed, and go to the station. I used to love to play all kinds of sports with my children, but now I would rather sit on the sofa than shoot hoops with my eight-year-old son or take a bicycle ride with my ten-year-old daughter. I am forgetting things at work and I doze off frequently when off camera. Add my weight gain to my poor performance and I wouldn't be surprised if my boss decided she wanted a younger, fitter, more with-it guy when my contract comes up for renewal. The worst thing is that I can't make myself care enough to show up differently.

It is not unusual for former athletes to lose their gusto and gain a gut as they get older. Testosterone plays a key role in body composition and fat cell metabolism. When levels begin to drop, men lose lean muscle mass and add on the pounds, particularly around the abdomen.

The change in body composition is more than cosmetic. Multiple studies show that men with low testosterone are at an increased risk of osteoporosis and fractures.[9] Lower testosterone levels are also associated with a loss of muscle mass and strength. The impact is much greater than simply a deterioration of a once muscle-bound physique. A 2007 report in the *Archives of Internal Medicine* found that men aged 65 to 99 with lower testosterone levels were more likely to fall than their counterparts with higher testosterone levels.[10]

While physical changes are obvious, testosterone's influence on emotional stability and cognition are subtle yet insidious. A 2008 study of approximately four thousand older men in Australia found that those with depression had significantly lower testosterone levels. In addition, several studies have shown that declining testosterone levels adversely affect memory and problem solving.[11]

When questioned about day-to-day life, many men report a loss of enthusiasm for simple joys, including family and hobbies. Others find it difficult to fully concentrate on tasks at work or at home. When combined with decreased libido and/or sexual performance issues, it is not uncommon for men to begin to question their manhood and identity in midlife. When a man comes into our practice complaining of fatigue, feeling low, and having a decreased sex drive, we see red flags waving. This man is in andropause.

Erectile Dysfunction: Much More Than Embarrassing

Let's get back to Rick's opening statement that he could no longer get it up. This is a common problem for men as they age. The 1994 Massachusetts Male Aging Study established erectile dysfunction (ED) as a plague stalking American men. Of 1,290 men aged 40 to 70 years, the combined prevalence of impotence was 52 percent. In 1998, former U.S. senator Bob Dole helped make ED the topic of everyday conversation when he honestly responded to a question about the aftermath of his prostate surgery on the *Larry King Show*. Producers of the segment said that their phone lines were immediately flooded with calls. Millions of men indicated that not only could they identify with the problem, they wanted help as well.

When you were in your 20s, you probably thought no more about getting a hard-on than you did about swallowing or urinating. Though seemingly effortless, your youthful erections resulted from a complex interplay among your nervous system, biologic activity, and hormones that begin when libido causes the sympathetic nervous system to release nitric oxide.

Nitric oxide causes the arteries to enlarge and blood to engorge the penis. A continual supply is essential for a firm, long-lasting erection. Both ED and heart disease have been linked with impaired nitric oxide activity, although struggles with erectile function usually precede symptoms of heart disease by several years. Release of nitric oxide can be sabotaged by elevated cholesterol levels, high blood pressure, increased triglycerides, smoking, metabolic syndrome, diabetes, and low testosterone levels. Because men with low testosterone are also at greater risk for heart disease, metabolic syndrome, and diabetes, the convergence amplifies the risk that optimum production of nitric oxide will be disrupted.

Are You in Andropause?

Men experience an age-related decline in DHEA production just as women do. According to the Massachusetts Male Aging Study, which investigated sexual function and activity in men aged 40 to 70, the incidence of ED increased as DHEA levels declined.[12]

Wondering whether your body is no longer producing enough testosterone or DHEA to fuel your sexual fires? If you are a man over 40 experiencing two or more of the following symptoms for three months or more, andropause is most likely why your life is increasingly limp and lustless:

- Decreased sex drive
- Decreased energy
- Decreased strength and endurance
- Erectile dysfunction
- Decreased sexual arousal and/or sensitivity
- Increased body fat
- Forgetfulness and difficulty concentrating
- Anxiety about sexual performance
- Decreased muscle mass
- Mild to moderate depression or irritability
- Feelings of loneliness
- Decrease in personal self-esteem
- Indecisiveness
- A reduction in sexual fantasies or frequency in masturbation
- Difficulty, or longer time frame for, recovering after working out
- Loss of enthusiasm for daily life
- Decreased work performance
- Increased lethargy
- More relationship problems and fights over sex, love, and intimacy

Wow. All those symptoms of declining hormone levels would cause any man to despair. Our good news is that andropause is not a terminal disease. Although you will never again be a 20-year-old stud, you can reclaim a hearty sex drive, a powerful erection, and a lean middle. The natural formula for restoring optimum testosterone levels and relieving erectile dysfunction varies from man to man. In Part Two you will learn about safe and effective options for hormone replacement. Part Three will then tell you the lifestyle choices—including diet, supplements, and exercise—that will keep you in the groove for good.

3

Other Hormone Balance and Sex Life Saboteurs

Age-related hormone imbalance is one culprit that steals your sex drive and pleasure, but there are others. Weight gain, chronic stress, and exposure to environmental estrogens, or xeno-estrogens, all disrupt hormone production. Subtle yet insidious, these sex life saboteurs run rampant in our lives. Their cumulative effect can be sexually stupefying.

Weight Gain Smothers Sex Drive

Walking into the reception of my thirty-five-year high school class reunion, I was stunned to see that two-thirds of my former classmates were more than pudgy—they were fat. I did not recognize Margo until I read her nametag. Previously a petite majorette with an hourglass figure, she was squeezed into a dress that had to be at least a size 16. Then there was Joey, an old crush and former football star, with a huge paunch spilling over his belt.

Susan, who used to be so skinny that her nickname was Flat-
bread, looked six months pregnant.

Big, soft bellies were my high school peer group's new common denominator. During my teenage years, a love of book reports and chemistry kept me out of the inner sanctum of the
fun-loving popular crowd. Once again, I was an outsider, but this
time it wasn't because I was a nerd; it was because I still had a
waist.

Over drinks and dinner, Margo turned the discussion my
way: "Genie, I hear you write books about hormones, health, and
sex. Since my divorce seven years ago, watching those hot doctors
on the television show *E.R.* is as sexy as I get. Do you have any
advice for a fat old lady like me?"

Brandon, whose once chiseled cleft chin was now flanked by
wobbly jowls, chimed in: "When we were kids, I was hot stuff. I
had some real steamy nights parked by the marina in my father's
old Lincoln. I thought the great thing about getting older would
be that you wouldn't have to sneak around and could have sex any
time you wanted. The irony is that now I have a great wife and a
king-size bed, but most nights the only thing I get up for is another beer."

Evelyn added her two cents: "I am afraid that reading your
new book would just make me feel guilty. My husband, Hank, is
always trying to get frisky. He doesn't care that I am 30 pounds
heavier than when we married, but I do. I mean, it's hard to feel
sexy when your body looks like a potato."

"Guys, you all have a point," I responded. "Being overweight
does affect your libido at a cellular level, but you can turn that
around. A few small changes can jump-start your sex drive."

"Tell us more," my old friends chorused.

My former classmates were in a big boat. According to a 2006 study published in the *Annals of Internal Medicine*, six out of ten Americans are overweight and about one in three is obese.[1] Obesity research shows that adults typically gain 1 to 2 pounds each year between the ages of 35 and 50—the same years defined by a significant age-related decline in hormone levels.[2]

Duke University doctors say two-thirds of obese people seeking treatment at the Duke Diet & Fitness Center report not enjoying or wanting to have sex, as well as having problems with sexual performance.[3] Randy and I observed an even higher correlation when conducting clinical research for our second book, *From Belly Fat to Belly Flat.* More than 85 percent of people seeking our help for hormone-related weight gain reported problems with sexual desire, performance, and/or pleasure.

Body fat is associated with poor body image and decreased sexual esteem. From a medical perspective, however, the inverse relationship of more weight to less sex can usually be traced to a coexisting hormone imbalance.

Estrogen Dominance, Your Big Belly, and Your Low Libido

Chapter 1 explained the link among estrogen dominance, low libido, and decreased sexual sensation in women. Body fat amplifies these sexual side effects.

Abdominal weight gain is one of the first symptoms of estrogen dominance. Pounds gravitate to the belly, butt, and thighs and won't budge, no matter how few calories you eat or how much you exercise. The worst part is that while age-related estrogen dominance causes weight gain, fat cells produce and store even more estrogen. The longer you have been overweight, the more likely you are to be caught in a vise of increasing estrogen dominance. Your fat cells continue to produce more estrogen, and your high estrogen levels cause you to continue to add more fatty tissue onto your body.

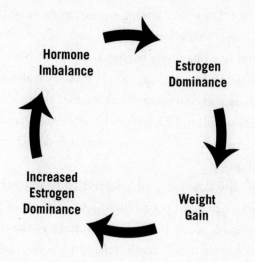

Increased estrogen dominance means that the symptoms will be more intense, including low libido, irritability, mood swings/depression, worsened PMS, headaches, hot flashes, night sweats, bloating, and foggy thinking. The more estrogen dominant you are, the more your body will resemble a potato and the less likely you are to ever feel in the mood again.

Estrogen dominance renders the thyroid hormones dysfunctional, causing metabolism to slow down. The resulting condition is called relative hypothyroidism. In addition to making it harder to burn calories and lose weight, hypothyroidism stimulates the production of prolactin, a hormone that interferes with the sex hormones, possibly lowering testosterone. The same thing occurs after childbirth. A surge in prolactin levels triggers milk production, but it also helps make sex about as appealing as a root canal to most new mothers.[4]

Testosterone Deficiency, Weight Gain, and Sexual Response

For men, the relationship among testosterone, weight gain, and sexual response is an intricate web. In Chapter 2, you learned how declining testosterone levels trigger a change in body composition, specifically a loss of lean muscle mass. You also read about how a deficiency in testosterone can increase the risk of medical conditions that lead to ED, such as heart disease, metabolic syndrome, and diabetes. Belly fat is another risk factor for these medical conditions.

Women also have sex problems related to testosterone deficiency, weight gain, and poor blood flow. "We are beginning to see that the width of the blood vessels leading to the clitoris [the area of the vagina most closely related to sexual response] in women is affected by the same kind of blockages that impact blood flow to the penis," says Susan Kellogg, director of sexual medicine at the Pelvic and Sexual Health Institute at the Graduate Hospital in Philadelphia. "When this happens, a woman's body is far less responsive, and a drop in desire is not far behind."[5]

Complicating matters further for both sexes, the more body fat you have, the higher your levels of sex hormone-binding globulin (SBGH). You learned in Chapter 1 how SBGH binds to testosterone like Velcro, leaving less available to stimulate desire. Body fat makes this chain of events even more sexually damning.

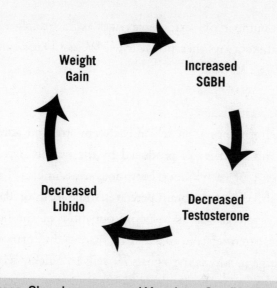

Stress, Sleeplessness, and Your Low-Sex/No-Sex Life

When Randy and I went to see the movie *Sex and the City*, I was particularly struck by the plight of one of the characters, Miranda, who is in her early 40s, healthy, and married to a man she loves. Though Miranda's husband craves her, Miranda goes six months or more without having or wanting sex.

If you haven't seen the movie, you might write Miranda off as an ice queen, but she isn't. She is juggling a full-time job, an hour commute to and from work, a small child, and a mother-in-law with Alzheimer's disease. Whenever her husband tries to initiate sex, she simply wants to get it over with so that she can get some much-needed sleep.

Miranda's situation is not unique. According to a 2007 study conducted by the American Psychological Association, 75 percent of Americans say they are too busy or too tired to have sex more than once a week.[6] Some psychologists estimate that 15 to 20 percent of working couples have sex no more than ten times a year. The number of sexless marriages is "a grossly underreported statistic," says therapist Michele Weiner Davis, author of *The Sex-Starved Marriage*.[7]

Too Stressed to Do It

The three hormones negatively impacted by stress are adrenaline, cortisol, and DHEA, all produced by the walnut-size adrenal glands on top of each kidney. How does stress impact these hormone levels? When the brain perceives some form of danger, it signals the adrenal glands to pump out more of the hormone adrenaline, often referred to as the flight-or-fight hormone. The sudden surge in adrenaline signals fat cells to quickly release energy. This energy rush stimulates flight, or running away.

Once the body is out of danger, the brain continues to signal the adrenal glands that there is a temporary need to keep adrenaline levels elevated. Higher than normal adrenaline levels cause an increase in appetite, which is needed to encourage the body to eat more calories and replenish fat stores. Under acute stress situations, adrenaline levels will soon return to normal once the immediate appetite has been satisfied.

This brain–body hormone-stimulating phenomenon served human beings very well in times when people were trying to avoid acute or immediate dangers, like the threat of being eaten by wolves or slaughtered by invading armies. Today, however, we are not usually subjected to such immediate dangers.

Contemporary stressors, like worrying about paying the mortgage, doing the jobs of three people, or grappling with ongoing parenting issues, tend to be more long term. A life stressor can be considered chronic if it persists for three or more months. Instead of pumping out more adrenaline, chronic stress causes the adrenal glands to secrete more of the hormone cortisol. Because chronic stress is ongoing, the adrenal glands can eventually become exhausted and unable to sustain cortisol production. A cortisol level that is too high or too low is a signal of chronic stress. Surveys find money and work to be the most common stresses associated with low-sex or no-sex relationships.[8]

Over time, elevated cortisol levels will wreak havoc on your sex life and your health. In addition to zapping your libido, sustained high cortisol levels destroy healthy muscle and bone, slow down healing and normal cell regeneration, co-opt biochemicals needed to make other vital hormones, impair digestion, dull mental processes, interfere with healthy endocrine function, and weaken your immune system. If you are stressed out, high cortisol levels will compromise your metabolism and cement more pounds around your middle, igniting the previously described cycle among body fat, estrogen dominance, testosterone level decline, and an even lower libido.

When the adrenals are chronically overworked and straining to maintain high cortisol levels, they lose the capacity to produce DHEA in sufficient amounts. You learned in Chapters 1 and 2 how DHEA promotes sexual appetite and response. When levels of DHEA are less than optimal, whether as a result of age-related decline or stressed-out adrenal glands, your sexuality is biochemically compromised.

Too Tired for Sex

Doctors have determined that lack of sleep slows sex drive. According to a 2005 National Sleep Foundation (NSF) nationwide poll of more than fifteen hundred respondents, 25 percent said they have sex less often or have lost interest in sex because they feel too sleepy. Another 25 percent said they forgo sex because of a snoring or constantly thrashing partner and, instead, choose to sleep in a separate bedroom.[9] Sleep, hormones, appetite, and sex function codependently. Consider the case of 45-year-old Bethany:

> Until a couple of years ago, my daily routine was to go to sleep around ten o'clock at night and have sex with my husband every morning minutes after our alarm went off. Now, because of my hot flashes and night sweats, we sleep in separate bedrooms. Not that I sleep much. Most nights, after tossing and turning for hours, I get up and make a sandwich or, worse, eat a sleeve of chocolate chip cookies. I am always hungry and increasingly sex-starved. What is wrong with me?

Bethany's age, hot flashes, night sweats, sleep disturbances, and low libido should lead you to believe she is estrogen dominant. In addition to too much estrogen, Bethany's sex life is being sabotaged by an imbalance between two other hormones produced by the hypothalamus: ghrelin and leptin. Ghrelin stimulates appetite; leptin signals the brain that you are full. Medical studies show that people who get less than eight hours of sleep a night have elevated ghrelin levels and suppressed leptin levels.

Bethany was up at night eating because an imbalance of ghrelin and leptin caused her to feel hungry regardless of how much she ate. With all those extra calories, more pounds would undoubtedly soon be packed around her middle. Bethany's situation illustrates how sleeplessness can further catalyze the previously described vicious cycle among body fat, estrogen dominance, testosterone deficiency, and less and less sex.

The Stealth Effect of Environmental Toxins

Mathew, a handsome 36-year-old, came to see us complaining of low libido and weak erections. His body weight was normal with a high percentage of lean muscle mass attributed to daily running and weight lifting. I began the consultation by asking Mathew a few questions about his stress level and lifestyle.

"I have a dream job," he said. "I run a family business that has been successful for decades. There is a great staff in place, which means I can take off whenever I want and still make money. I am newly married to a smart, beautiful woman named Hannah. My only real stress is that our sex life is almost nonexistent, and it is all my fault. Before we married, Hannah would say, 'I would rather be with a man who loves my mind,' but now she tells me she wants a baby, which means we have to have sex, which means I have to perform." Mathew's voice trailed off despairingly.

Here was a fit, relatively young man with no work or money stressors married to a woman who he adored. So, what was keeping him from being raring to go? I probed more about his job.

"My grandfather started our family's dry-cleaning business. I worked with him from the time I was 8 years old and never stopped. We were opening three new storefronts when I graduated from high school, so I stayed home to help and took college courses at night. My grandfather passed away years ago and my father recently retired. Now it is all on my shoulders, but that's okay. I'm up for it," Mathew concluded with a smile.

You may be up for your work, I thought, but being exposed to dry-cleaning fumes for decades is the most likely reason you are not up for sex.

Environmental estrogens, or xenoestrogens, are prolific in

our everyday lives. They can be found in certain pesticides, herbicides, fungicides, plastics, fuels, car exhaust, dry-cleaning chemicals, industrial waste, meat from livestock fed estrogenic drugs to fatten them up, lawn care solutions, and hair products. Even that "healthy" plastic bottle of water you carry around can leach xenoestrogens from the plastic into the water, depositing them into your system upon drinking.

We are also exposed to synthetic estrogens and synthetic progesterone (chemically termed *progestin*) because of the millions of women taking birth-control pills and synthetic hormone therapies. These xenohormones filter into the urine and get flushed down the toilet. Unfortunately, they are not filtered out by water and sewage plants, so they eventually make their way back into the food chain.

Fifty-one chemicals have now been identified as hormone disrupters, at least half of which resist the natural processes of decay, some persisting for decades, some for centuries. Over time, these foreign estrogens can dangerously accumulate and increase

> Chemical compounds ubiquitous in our food, air, and water are now found in every person. The bioaccumulation of these compounds in some individuals can lead to a variety of metabolic and systemic dysfunctions, and in some cases outright disease states. The systems most affected by these xenoestrogen compounds include the immune, neurological, and endocrine systems. Toxicity in these systems can lead to immune dysfunction, autoimmunity, asthma, allergies, cancers, cognitive deficit, mood changes, neurological illnesses, changes in libido, reproductive dysfunction, and glucose dysregulation.
>
> —*Alternative Medicine Review* 5(1) (2000): 52–63.

the estrogen load in the body, contributing to early puberty and many significant health risks for adults. Loss of libido is just one of the casualties.

Multiple research studies in the United States and Europe show a link between xenoestrogens, particularly estrogenic steroids used to fatten livestock, and an increased incidence of prostate and breast cancers. Other studies cite xenoestrogens as the culprit contributing to an increased incidence of testicular cancer, decreased sperm counts, volume of sperm ejaculated, unhealthy sperm, and reproductive abnormalities.[10]

Misdiagnosis and Medications Kill Your Libido

Harriet and Donovan are a happily married couple in their early 50s. Fourteen months before we met, they had attended a sacred sex weekend hosted by their church.

"After that, our sex lives got worse instead of better," Harriet told me. "When we shared that we were still very much in love after twenty-seven years of marriage but that we only had sex every month or so, our pastor told us, 'People in love want to have sex. They shouldn't go one week without it.' He was very concerned that we might both be suffering from depression and counseled us to see a doctor. That really shook me up, because with the kids happily away at college, I felt lighter and more excited about my life than I had in years. I hadn't really thought our minimal sex life could be anything more than a symptom of getting older."

Donovan injected, "I didn't feel depressed, either, but I did miss having a more active sex life, so I told Harriet perhaps we should get things checked out. We saw our family physician, but he wasn't in the room with us two minutes before he started writing prescriptions. Harriet got one for Prozac and I got one for Viagra."

"I feel much worse instead of better," said Harriet. "I have gained 20 pounds, have frequent migraines, and the idea of having sex is about as appealing as a tour of the city sewer plant."

"How about you?" I asked Donovan.

"Erections were never my problem, so I didn't even fill that prescription for Viagra. Even if Harriet's prescription had helped her get in the mood again, my problem is that I am never in the mood, and I guess I will continue to feel this way from here on out. Now that is really depressing."

Well-intentioned physicians frequently misdiagnose and mistreat symptoms of hormone imbalance. Many of the drugs prescribed as symptom band-aids will further compromise libido. For instance, a woman or a man with an underlying hormone imbalance who complains of mood swings and lethargy is likely to be misdiagnosed and prescribed an antidepressant. Selective serotonin reuptake inhibitors (SSRIs), such as Prozac, Lexapro, and Paxil, are a frequently prescribed group of antidepressants clinically associated with a decrease in sex drive.

The synthetic hormones in birth-control pills also hamper libido. "Lots of women on the birth-control pill complain of a lower sex drive," says gynecologist Christine Derzko, an author on sexual dysfunction and an associate professor of obstetrics and gynecology at the University of Toronto. "The [synthetic] estrogen in the pill increases the amount of binding globulins in the blood, which mop up the free testosterone that's floating around."[11] As you will learn in Chapter 4, loss of libido is only one of the health dangers associated with synthetic hormones.

Sedatives or tranquilizers such as Valium, Librium, and

Xanax can cause sexual side effects in men and women. They are part of a group of drugs that act on the limbic area of the brain by relaxing the connection between the sensory and motor pathways. This allows the skeletal muscles to relax. Libido is diminished and sexual response slackens.

Many over-the-counter drugs cause sexual side effects. Medicines for colds, coughs, and allergies that cause drowsiness can affect sex drive. Another common side effect is a decrease in lubrication. Antiulcer drugs like Tagamet that work to block the secretion of stomach acid have caused impotence in men because they can block peripheral testosterone receptors. Diuretics taken for bloating can negatively affect the libido. Nonsteroidal anti-inflammatory drugs (NSAIDs), such as the popular Advil and Motrin, often make it difficult for people to reach full arousal and can cause a reduction of natural lubrication.

Multiple drugs with similar side effects can cumulatively kill your libido. Too often doctors and pharmacists neglect to inform you about the sexual side effects of some drugs. If you think medication might be dulling your desire, read package inserts and find out whether you have other treatment options.

When Men Sit and Women Bitch, Sex Gets Sidelined

Pick up any book or magazine article discussing women, relationships, and sex and you will read about how women want more intimacy before they want more sex. In her book *Real Sex for Real Women*, Laura Berman states, "In a healthy long-term relationship, men and women are fortunate to have a lover who is also their best friend. Sex and romance are crucial for long-term intimacy."[12]

In the surveys of women I conducted while writing this

book, the consensus was that feeling emotionally connected and genuinely loved was as important—if not more so—than having an orgasm. Most women state that good, open, and regular communication is required to feel emotionally connected. Regrettably, an underlying hormone imbalance can throw a wrench in both healthy communication styles and sexual desire for both sexes. Consider the case of 43-year-old Meaghen and 48-year-old David. First, Meaghen shares her point of view:

> David and I used to enjoy catching up while our children did their homework and we prepared dinner. That time talking together was my favorite hour of the day. Each time I shared and he listened, I would fall in love all over again. And when David would roll up his sleeves to cut vegetables or do dishes, I would look at his biceps and start fantasizing about the rest of his body. As the evening progressed, I would get increasingly turned on. By the time we were alone in bed, I would be revved up and ready to go.
>
> Now, David comes in, pours himself a glass of wine, and flops his increasingly big butt on the sofa, saying, "I am too tired to help out with dinner," as if he was the only one with a demanding job. I come home from my office feeling completely wiped out, often with an excruciating headache, but I still make our evening meal, do a couple of loads of laundry, and help the children with their studies. David just sits and stares at the television. He moans and groans if I insist he do the smallest thing, like taking out the garbage or walking the dog. If he reaches for me in bed, I get angry. I used to have a partner that would talk, laugh, and make love to me. Now, he just wants to use our home—and me—as a pit stop.

Here's David's take on the situation:

Meaghen and I have been married for nineteen years. I first fell in love with her because she was more gentle, kind, and giving than any girl I had ever met. She always made an extra effort to say things to make me feel good. "You are the best husband in the world," she would say, or, "I am so proud of the way you take care of our family."

In the last few years, however, Meaghen has changed. Now, all she can talk about is how lazy I am or how fat I am getting. I haven't told her about how younger men at the office are getting promoted over me because I can't keep up the workload I used to. I am afraid she would ridicule rather than comfort me. I don't have much of a sex drive anymore and can only seem to get an erection in the morning, but I miss how I used to hold Meaghen until we fell asleep. Sometimes I reach out to cuddle, but it is usually a lost cause. The last time I tried, she launched into a tirade, telling me, "I am more than a sex kitten." "That's for sure," I told her. "Kittens don't have fangs."

Here is an excerpt of my notes following both interviews:

Meaghen: 43 years old, premenopausal

Irritability

Fatigue

Headaches

Low libido

Probable diagnosis: age-related estrogen dominance compounded by stress-induced elevated cortisol levels

David: 48 years old, andropausal

Fatigue/lethargy

Depression

Weight gain

Deteriorating work performance

Low libido

Erectile performance issues

Probable diagnosis: significant decline in testosterone

levels

Can you see how symptoms of hormone imbalance were sabotaging Meaghen and David's communication as well as their sexual intimacy? Can you identify?

Is Your Life Contributing to Your Sexual Problems?

If you answer yes to any of the following five questions, a variable other than age is increasing your risk of hormone imbalance and contributing to your sexual problems:

1. Have you been 10 pounds or more overweight for more than a year?
2. Have you been attempting to cope with a stressful situation or event for more than three months? This might include divorce, relationship problems, angry teenagers, aging parents, work stress, job worries, financial problems, and anything else that makes you feel tense, anxious, or constantly worried.
3. Do you work more than 40 hours a week?

4. Do you sleep less than eight hours a night?
5. Do you live in the United States or another industrialized nation awash in xenoestrogens?

The good news is that you can stop these sex life saboteurs dead in their tracks.

Part Two:

Hormone Replacement Can Turn Up the Heat, . . . But Don't Get Burned

You are now convinced that hormones, or lack of, are responsible for your low libido. It seems reasonable that you could once again have the sex drive of your youth if only you could restore your body's optimum hormone balance. But is that medically possible? And what about side effects and health risks? Part Two provides the answers to these questions and more.

Chapter 4 describes why pharmaceutically manufactured synthetic hormones are very risky. You will learn how drug manufacturers first launched hormone replacement therapy (HRT) drugs, such as the popular Premarin, as the female fountain of youth even though medical evidence of their carcinogenic properties was already on the table. More recent medical research studies have not only linked HRT to an increased risk of cancer but also to an increased risk of heart disease, stroke, blood clots, and Alzheimer's. Already wondering why these dangerous drugs remain on the market? Chapter 4 goes behind the scenes to give you the inside scoop.

Chapter 5 clearly establishes bioidentical hormone replacement therapy (BHRT) as a medically sound option for reestablishing optimum hormone levels and rejuvenating your sex drive. This chapter expounds on the fundamental premise of BHRT that one size does not fit all by explaining how your personal hormone-level profile is obtained and why it is needed. It then describes how age-related hormone-level decline manifests differently for women and men.

Chapter 6 explains why BHRT is a wonderful option for restoring hormone balance and rejuvenating your sex drive, but it is not a panacea for all. Because conventional physicians have been slow to adopt BHRT as a first-line treatment for symptoms of hormone imbalance, you may have difficulty locating a medical expert who is qualified to prescribe it. Also, BHRT can be expensive. We help you sort through controversial approaches and also shed light on why some pharmaceutical companies continue to oppose the dispensing of personalized BHRT prescriptions.

4

The Dangers of Synthetic Hormone Replacement Therapy

In 1942, Ayerst Labs financed the market launch of America's first synthetic hormone replacement therapy (HRT) drug. Ayerst's marketing geniuses aptly named the drug Premarin, as it was a blend of conjugated estrogens extracted from the urine of pregnant mares. Doctors across the country were grateful to finally have an option for effectively helping women suffering from menopausal symptoms, such as hot flashes, night sweats, moodiness, and low libido.

Women were excited that modern science had formulated a hormone replacement fountain of youth. Upscale magazine advertisements purported that with this product you could now circumvent a formerly inevitable fate of becoming a dried-up, increasingly unattractive, and witchy old woman. Not surprisingly, the market demand for Premarin skyrocketed.

Fast forward sixty years. It was 2002 and the Premarin family of products had become a $2.07 billion industry for Wyeth, the pharmaceutical manufacturer.[1] But wait! The government-funded Women's Health Initiative (WHI) study on HRT was brought to a screeching halt in July 2002 when a safety monitoring board determined that women taking Prempro (a combination of Premarin and synthetic progesterone or progestin) experienced a significantly increased risk of breast and uterine cancers, heart attack, stroke, blood clots, and Alzheimer's disease.

Word hit the streets immediately through newspapers, television, and radio. Women were frightened, and more than 50 percent of those taking synthetic hormone products immediately stopped their prescriptions. As a direct result of the WHI findings, Wyeth's revenues from the Premarin family of products declined by more than 57 percent in only three years, from $2.07 billion in 2001 to $880 million in 2004. In 2005, an ongoing decline in sales of these drugs caused the drug maker to announce the closing of its manufacturing plant in Rouses, New York, and the phasing out of twelve hundred jobs.

Now, the Premarin drugs are back, but in a slightly different formulation. Wyeth is pumping millions of dollars into marketing its new low-dose hormone therapy, Prempro 0.45 mg/1.5 mg, which contains 28 percent less synthetic estrogen and 40 percent less progestin. "Go low with Prempro" TV spots and magazine ads urge female consumers. Coincidently, Wyeth's leagues of sales representatives visit physician offices armed with marketing materials and lunch. The impact: Many conventional physicians once again feel safe choosing this synthetic hormone cocktail as their first line of treatment for women suffering from menopausal symptoms.

Still, controversy abounds. Wyeth is being sued by women in multiple states who claim they got breast cancer because they took Premarin or Prempro. The integrity of Wyeth's medical research is also under scrutiny. A December 2008 article published in the *Wall Street Journal* reported that Senator Charles Grassley of Iowa has launched a Senate investigation to determine if the pharmaceutical giant paid ghostwriters to pen medical journal articles falsely downplaying the link between synthetic hormone replacement therapies, specifically Prempro, and breast cancer risk.[2] Ghostwriting is a practice in which manuscripts are written or heavily developed by others, including marketing specialists, to contain a spin on the information beyond the scope of what has been written by the medical scientists named as the primary authors. As Randy and I first said in *From Hormone Hell to Hormone Well*, "When marketing gets ahead of science, the health of innocent people can suffer."

Because of the cacophony of dissenting information, many people remain legitimately confused and frightened regarding their options and who they should trust for guidance. What is the real story?

The Horror of the First Synthetic Hormone Studies

Some of the first scientific experiments with synthetic hormones were conducted in Germany during World War II. The Schering pharmaceutical company paid a biochemist named Adolph Friedrich Johann Butenandt to use women in Auschwitz as guinea pigs for testing synthetic hormones as a form of birth control.[3] The goal of these experiments was to sterilize the Jews so that they would not be able to perpetuate their race, but while still alive could serve as slave laborers for the "superior" Aryan race.[4] Butenandt ordered that the Jewish women unknowingly be fed high doses of synthetic estrogen in their daily servings of ruta-baga soup.

Butenandt's experiments were unsuccessful. Women in Auschwitz continued to have offspring. Still, there was heinous damage, and the ripple effect would be felt for generations. Decades later, testing of hundreds of children of Holocaust survivors would show that the Auschwitz contingent had the lowest IQ range. Medical researchers postulated that the synthetic hormone experiments were responsible.[5]

Why Are Synthetic Hormones Dangerous?

When used to describe hormones, the terms *synthetic* and *natural* can often be confusing. Synthetic hormones have a molecular structure that has been chemically altered to be different from the hormones produced by the human body. Why are they chemically altered to have a different molecular structure? It is all about profit. Pharmaceutical companies cannot patent a molecular structure found in nature. By altering the molecular structure of the hormone, the pharmaceutical manufacturer can have exclusive ownership of both the chemical formula and the revenue generated by its synthetic hormone product until its patent expires.

Consider the hormones produced within your body to be unique keys fitting into specific hormone receptor locks throughout your body, including the brain. When the hormone receptor lock recognizes and receives its unique key, it smoothly "unlocks" its specific function, whether that is growth and maturation, libido, energy, metabolism, or cognitive function. The biochemical term for this perfect fit is *relative binding affinity (RBA)*. All hormones produced within the human body have a 100 percent RBA for their corresponding hormone receptor lock.

When the molecular structure of the hormone has been altered, as is the case with synthetic hormones, it does not fit perfectly into your body's hormone receptor locks. Even a slight variation can trigger a negative reaction at a cellular level, ultimately causing side effects, some uncomfortable and others potentially lethal. Consider the difference between progesterone produced by the ovaries and pharmaceutically manufactured synthetic progestin.

When pregnant, the female body needs its progesterone to support and nurture the fetus. The RBA for the progesterone produced within the body is 100 percent. If progestin—with its slightly altered molecular structure and reduced RBA of only 78 percent—were to be given to a pregnant woman, she would either miscarry or the baby would suffer fetal abnormalities.

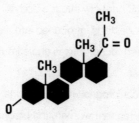

Progesterone

Relative Binding Affinity = 100

Source: Human Pharmacology, 3rd ed, Mosby-Year Book, Inc. (1998).

The human body possesses progesterone receptors throughout almost all body tissues. The progesterone produced by a woman's ovaries fits perfectly into its receptor as nature intended and elicits the appropriate response.

In pregnancy, the corpus luteum secretes progesterone to support the maturation of the fetus for about ten to twelve weeks, or until the placenta is large enough to take over. If a pregnancy is at risk during the first trimester, bioidentical progesterone is prescribed to help the body to continue to support the fetus and bring the pregnancy to term.

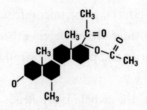

Progestin (medroxyprogesterone acetate)

Relative Binding Affinity = 78

Source: C. W. Randolph, Jr. (May 2009). *From Hormone Hell to Hormone Well,* 2009, p. 26.

The human body does not possess receptors for progestins (synthetic progesterone). Progestin's RBA is only 78 percent, meaning that this synthetic molecule key does not fit perfectly into the body's hormone receptor locks. Biochemically, when progestin is introduced into the human system, it confuses the body's cells and receptor sites and stimulates a negative and defensive immune response.

Whereas bioidentical progesterone supports pregnancy, if progestin was administered to a pregnant woman, the pregnancy would be compromised, and if the fetus survived, it would have a significantly higher risk for fetal abnormalities (birth defects).

Now consider Premarin: a "natural" mixture of estrogens made by a biological organism, a pregnant mare. But, as the late Dr. John Lee, one of the pioneers in the field of bioidentical hormone replacement, would say, "The estrogens in Premarin are only 'natural' if your favorite food is hay."

The types of estrogen that make up Premarin do not exist in

the human body. Therefore, when introduced into the human system, their partial fit into the body's hormone receptor locks triggers side effects at a cellular level. In addition to WHI's momentous findings, in 2007 the *New England Journal of Medicine* published powerful evidence linking the significant drop in breast cancer rates to the sharp drop in synthetic hormone use by menopausal women.[6] Unfortunately for those women who participated in WHI, a 2008 study published in the *Journal of the American Medical Association (JAMA)* reported that three years after stopping their drugs, women who had taken the synthetic estrogen plus progestin combo drug Prempro during the WHI trials had a 27 percent higher risk of developing breast cancer than those in the trial who took the placebo.[7]

In the United States, a black box warning appears on the package insert for prescription drugs that may cause serious or even life-threatening adverse effects. It is so named because a black border surrounds the text of the warning. The Food and Drug Administration (FDA) can require a pharmaceutical company to place a back box warning on the labeling of a prescription drug or in the literature describing it. It is the strongest warning required by the FDA. Here is the black box warning included in the package insert for the Premarin family of drugs:

What is the most important information you should know about PREMARIN (estrogens), PREMPRO (a combination of estrogens and a progestin), or PREMARIN Vaginal Cream (a cream of estrogens)?

- Estrogens increase the chance of getting cancer of the uterus. Report any unusual vaginal bleeding right away while you are using these products. Vaginal bleeding after menopause may be a warning sign of cancer of the uterus (womb). Your health care provider should check any unusual vaginal bleeding to find out the cause.

- Do not use estrogens with or without progestins to prevent heart disease, heart attacks, strokes, or dementia.

Using estrogens, with or without progestins, may increase your chance of getting heart attacks, strokes, breast cancer, and blood clots. Using estrogens, with or without progestins, may increase your chance of getting dementia, based on a study of women age 65 years or older. You and your health care provider should talk regularly about whether you still need treatment with estrogens.

This section has focused on a discussion of the dangers of the Premarin family of products because they were the specific synthetic hormone drugs used in the WHI study and they are the synthetic hormones that have been most popularly prescribed. Although other synthetic hormone products do not have the largesse of market share, they share the same health risks. Brand names include FemHRT, Activella, Ortho-Prefest, CombiPatch, Cenestin, Menest, Ortho-Est, Ogen, and Estratab.

What About the Pill?

When Ellen walked into my office, I did a double-take. This 48-year-old mother and advertising executive could have walked away with a prize in a Nicole Kidman look-alike contest.

"Genie, I am confused," she began. "I have been on the Pill for nine years. I like the convenience, and my PMS symptoms are much better when I am on it, but recently I read in a women's magazine that the Pill can depress sex drive. A lightbulb went off in my head. I used to love sex during the years I was getting pregnant and having babies, but since my doctor put me on the Pill, I would rather clean out my e-mail inbox than get naked and go for it. I talked to my doctor about evaluating other options for contraception, but she told me, 'The Pill helps keep you young. Your skin won't wrinkle and your vagina will be as moist and ready as a teenager's.' What do you think?"

I told Ellen that I feared she and her doctor were victims of a pharmaceutical marketing department snow-job.

As described in Chapter 3, birth-control pills contain synthetic estrogen and synthetic progesterone. In addition to their proven dampening effect on sex drive, long-term use of birth-control pills can be a health hazard. Depending on dosage, they can be very potent and linger for a long period in the body. Birth-control pills work by keeping estrogen at such a falsely high level that the body is fooled into thinking it is pregnant. Therefore, ovulation does not occur.

Fears about blood clots, heart attack, and stroke, which spurred exhaustive research in the 1960s and 1970s, have for the most part been laid to rest by the safer, low-dose birth-control pills on the market today. Questions about the Pill's association with cancer remain. According to the Women's Lifestyle and Health Study, one of the largest international studies on oral contraception use, women over 45 using the Pill are one-and-a-half times more likely to get breast cancer as women who never used the Pill.[8] If you are currently taking the Pill or considering it as a means of contraception, research and evaluate your options.

If you have had all the children you desire or do not desire children, there are three other options. You can have a surgical tubal ligation (having your tubes tied), or your partner/husband can have a vasectomy. A newer technique is to have your tubes occluded. This minimally invasive procedure, called Essure, can be done in a medical office or outpatient facility. A scope is placed through the vagina and cervix into the uterus, and plugs are inserted into the tubal openings. Essure requires minimal recovery and no incisions. It takes approximately ten minutes and is five times more effective than having your tubes tied. A downside to this technique is that it takes three months for the plugs to grow into the openings for total occlusion of the fallopian tubes. During this window of time, an alternate method of birth control should be used.

If you want to postpone pregnancy, you may consider condoms, an intrauterine device (IUD), cervical caps, a diaphragm, withdrawal, spermicide, or the Billings ovulation method—a natural method that women can use to monitor fertility based on sensation in the vulva and the appearance and consistency of vaginal mucus discharge. According to the World Health Organization, the Billings ovulation method is 99.5 percent effective in postponing pregnancy when followed correctly.[9]

So What's a Girl Supposed to Do?

You are burning up with hot flashes, you haven't slept through the night in months, and the idea of sex is unappealing. You know it's your hormones and you go to your doctor for help. He or she wants to write you a prescription for a synthetic hormone drug. You are desperate for relief, but you are also scared of the long-term health consequences. What should you do?

First and foremost, take responsibility for your own health. Long gone is the era when our parents regarded their physicians as "MD-ieties"—the all-knowing sources of irrefutable health care information. As smart and well intentioned as your doctor might be, you have the ultimate say regarding what medications you do or do not take.

Next, do your homework. As you will soon learn, synthetic hormones are only one option for treating symptoms of hormone imbalance. Both BHRT and our three-step approach to naturally boosting lagging hormone levels are safe and effective alternatives that will not only relieve your symptoms but will also positively impact your health. Do your own research. Use the Internet and/or get a second opinion from a holistic medical professional. Then decide for yourself whether our position is medically valid.

If, after you have evaluated all options, you decide that taking a synthetic hormone replacement drug is best for you, we respect your decision but also urge you to be both cautious and vigilant. Take the lowest dose for the shortest possible period of time, be on the alert for side effects, and stop immediately if any should occur. In the beginning, these side effects might be subtle—such as weight gain, headaches, foggy thinking, or decreased sex drive—but they should be regarded as an immediate red flag. As Randy says, "A little less poison is still poison. If you are allergic to shellfish, eating only one or eating a dozen shrimp will both put you in anaphylactic shock."

Bioidentical Hormone Replacement Therapy: A Safe and Effective Alternative

Randy and I receive daily e-mails and telephone calls from women and men taking the initiative to learn more about options for hormone replacement. Many are concerned about the side effects associated with synthetic HRT and wonder whether bioidentical hormone replacement therapy (BHRT) might be a safer alternative, but they are confused. Here are some of the most frequently asked questions:

- "I watched Oprah's television shows on hormone replacement, but I still don't understand," says Trina. "Exactly what are bioidentical hormones? Why are they different from synthetic hormones if they are also made in a laboratory?"

- "I saw a hormone cream in a health food store that was labeled bioidentical," Paul reports. "But I thought bioidentical hormones required a prescription. Are they also available over the counter, and, if so, what is the difference between

the ones I might buy in a health food store and the ones my
doctor would prescribe?"

- Martha writes in an e-mail: "In one of your books, Dr.
  Randolph states, 'An advantage of BHRT is that one size
  does not fit all.' What exactly does that mean?"
- Britney wants to know: "If bioidentical hormones are just like
  the ones my body makes, where do they come from?"
- "I already take a Mexican wild yam supplement for my hot
  flashes. That is natural, right? Is it also bioidentical?" Elisha
  asks.
- "My internist told me that BHRT has been under fire by the
  Federal Drug Administration," Stanley tells me. "What's the
  deal with that?"

Wondering whether BHRT could be your sexual salvation?
We'll explain the difference between BHRT and synthetic hormones, some basic BHRT formulations you can procure over the
counter (and when it's best to see a doctor), what to ask your
doctor for in a hormone-level profile, and most important, how
to stay safe and healthy while you're using BHRT.

What Is BHRT and Why Is It Safe?

Randy has used BHRT as his first-line treatment for thousands
of women and men suffering from hormone-related sexual dysfunction for more than a decade; however, he did not always prescribe BHRT. Like most physicians in the United States, Randy
was trained in medical school to prescribe synthetic HRT, so for
several years after opening his medical practice, he did. He
stopped because of the high percentage of patients who came

back complaining of side effects: some troublesome, like low libido and weight gain; others of greater health significance, like tender or fibrocystic breasts. Years before the Women's Health Initiative tagged HRT as a health risk, Randy researched a safer alternative. His experience as a compounding pharmacist combined with his intensive studies in the biochemistry of plant-based medicine helped him recognize BHRT as a spot-on mechanism for restoring hormone balance at a cellular level. Here's why:

Bioidentical hormones are synthesized in a laboratory from plant precursor molecules called diosgenins that are found in Mexican wild yam and soy. The goal is to ensure that bioidentical hormones have exactly the same molecular structure as the hormones produced by the human body. They are often referred to as "natural" because the body's hormone receptor locks recognize and receive bioidentical hormones in the same way as hormones produced by the ovaries, testes, adrenal glands, and hypothalamus. Thus, they do not trigger side effects. Bioidentical hormones are safe because, like the hormones produced by your body, they have a 100 percent relative binding affinity (RBA) for your internal hormone receptor sites.

Do I Need to See a Doctor to Get BHRT?

Medical research has proven that when BHRT is used to reestablish the body's optimum hormone levels, good things happen at a cellular level. Which bioidentical hormone and how much of it you need will depend on your individual physiology. The objective of BHRT is to replace deficient hormones in order to restore optimum hormone balance. Because you are an individual with a unique composite of hormone activity, your specific hormones and dosages will most likely be very different from what your best friend, neighbor, or sister might need. As we'll discuss later in the chapter, there are some times when over-the-counter bio-identical hormone formulations will provide significant relief from hormone imbalance, and in other situations a doctor may be needed to prescribe a personalized formulation prepared by a compounding pharmacist. Consider Paula and Meredith's story:

As colleagues in an advertising agency, Paula and Meredith frequently traveled together for business. At 53, Meredith was fit and energetic with a sexual aura that caused men's heads to turn whenever she walked into a room. She often entertained Paula with stories of her many suitors and their weekend trysts.

"How do you manage to balance this job, an active love life, and still have the energy to work out three times a week?" queried 37-year-old Paula. "By the time I get home, all I want to do is have a glass of wine, get in the bathtub, and go to bed and sleep. No sex, just sleep. What is your secret?"

"Paula, I have been taking bioidentical hormones for seven years now. It is as if they have turned back a clock within my body. Honestly, I feel more alive and have more sexual vitality than I did at your age," Meredith confided.

"Can I try your prescription while we are on this trip?" Paula asked hopefully. "If they work, my husband will be so grateful and I'll make an appointment with my doctor next week."

"Honey, my BHRT prescription has been formulated just for me. The prescription of BHRT that a young girl like you would need would be very different than one that works for a menopausal woman like me," Meredith explained.

A key premise of prescription BHRT is that one size does

not fit all. A premenopausal woman like Paula will have a very different hormone-level profile than a woman who has already gone through menopause. Meredith's personalized BHRT prescription had been prescribed by a physician after a full battery of hormone-level tests determined which hormones were lacking in her body. As a woman in menopause for several years, Meredith required a BHRT formulation of all three sex hormones to restore optimum hormone balance. Paula, in contrast, was starting to experience some premenopausal hormone fluctuations, indicating that her progesterone levels were beginning to drop. A woman with this concern will often find that an over-the-counter formulation could be the answer.

Over-the-Counter BHRT Formulations

If you are a woman, you already know that each age and stage of life brings with it unique joys and challenges, from motherhood to career maven to wisdom bearer. It should not be a surprise that your path of hormone replacement will also become multifactorial as the years go by. The mix and amount of bioidentical hormones required to restore optimum hormone balance in your 30s will be different in your 40s and 50s.

Bioidentical Progesterone: A Lifetime Player

Because female progesterone levels are the first to decline, many younger women find that bioidentical progesterone is all they need to get their mojo back in gear. Consider 41-year-old Piper's experience:

> I am normally an easygoing person, but after I turned 40, I found myself constantly snapping at the kids, yelling at my husband, and getting angry in traffic. I didn't realize how my sex drive had

evaporated until my husband complained that I was "always hot under the collar during the day, but I was nothing but a cold shoulder under the covers at night."

A friend suggested I try bioidentical progesterone cream. I didn't have much faith that some cream would help very much, but boy was I surprised. In less than two weeks, I was my old calm and patient self. I could once again take my rambunctious teenagers in stride. I was humming while driving and—according to my husband—I was back to making things hum in our bedroom as well.

In these early years of hormone production decline, many women can self-treat an underlying progesterone deficiency with an over-the-counter bioidentical progesterone cream available in most health food stores or over the Internet. Bioidentical progesterone is very safe and side effects are rare. The most common side effect is drowsiness.

The concentration of bioidentical progesterone in an over-the-counter cream is less than the percentage in an individualized prescription formulation. The good news is that these creams are easily available. The bad news is that you don't always know what you are getting. Most product labels do not answer the following questions:

- Is the progesterone truly bioidentical?
- Do the hormones used in the formulation meet the U.S. Pharmacopoeia gold standards for quality and purity?
- Was the progesterone product actually compounded under the strict guidelines approved by the National Association of Compounding Pharmacists?
- Will the type of oil in the cream formulation promote or inhibit transdermal absorption?

Dr. Randolph's Natural Balance Cream meets the highest quality standards and is available through our Web site: www .hormonewell.com. In addition, a listing of other over-the-counter bioidentical progesterone creams that Randy has scrutinized for quality and safety is included in Appendix B.

Follow package directions when using any over-the-counter product; however, if not noted, always apply bioidentical progesterone cream above the waist. A recent Australian study showed that transdermal progesterone applied below the waist or on the legs can get into the liver through collateral circulation. This liver pass-through effect decreases effectiveness. Also, it is important to rotate the application site of bioidentical progesterone cream.

No matter how your prescription for BHRT may change over the years, bioidentical progesterone should remain a lifetime player in every woman's personal regimen of bioidentical hormone replacement. In addition to its uplifting effect on

---

Dr. Randolph's Natural Balance Cream
Application Instructions

Apply cream twice daily, morning and evening, to the area marked "1" in the figure. The next day, choose another numbered area and apply twice daily to that area. Continue rotating the site of cream application, moving to another numbered area each day. Repeat rotation of cream application sites.

Always use progesterone cream twice daily. Using progesterone cream alone is safe.

Caution: If you still have your uterus, do not take estrogen without progesterone. This may cause precancerous cells to form in the uterine lining.

Special Instructions:

PMS: Use 1 to 2 pumps twice a day from days 8–26 of your cycle.

Osteoporosis: Use 1 to 2 pumps twice a day for 25 days, and then take 5 days off. Repeat. After 3 months, decrease to ½ to 1 pump twice a day. If using with estrogen, use every day of the month.

Endometriosis: Use 2 pumps twice a day from days 6–26 of your cycle.

Ovarian Cysts: Use 1 to 2 pumps twice a day from days 8–26 of your cycle.

Fibrocystic Breasts: Use 1 to 2 pumps twice a day from days 8–26 of your cycle.

Uterine Fibroids: Use 1 to 2 pumps twice a day from days 8–26 of your cycle.

Pre- or Perimenopause: Use 1 to 2 pumps twice a day from days 8–26 of your cycle. If using with estrogen, use every day of the month.

Postmenopsause or Hysterectomy: Use 1 to 2 pumps twice a day for 25 days. Then take 5 days off. Repeat. After 3 months, decrease to 1 pump twice a day. If using with estrogen, use every day of the month.

Men: 45 years and older, use ⅛ teaspoon or 1 pump twice a day.

Application Areas: 1 = right forearm; 2 = right breast; 3 = chest; 4 = left breast; 5 = left forearm; 6 = neck.

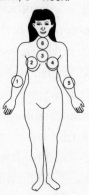

Note: First day of bleeding is the first day of your cycle. If you have additional questions, visit www.hormonewell.com.

libido and calming effect on moods, clinical studies demonstrate that bioidentical progesterone can eliminate PMS and menopausal symptoms, including hot flashes, anxiety, sleep disturbances, and mood swings. And, when optimum equilibrium between estrogen and progesterone levels is restored, cardiovascular health, nervous system function, and bone health are also improved.

Medical research exploring the potential breast cancer–protective properties of bioidentical progesterone is gaining attention across the globe. In Chapter 1, you learned how estrogen stimulates cell growth and how unchecked cell growth can lead to cancer when the body is estrogen dominant. Introducing bioidentical progesterone into the body halts this cellular overgrowth. In 2005, a groundbreaking study published in the *International Journal of Cancer* showed that bioidentical progesterone could decrease breast cancer risk by 10 percent. Other studies show a decrease of 20 percent or more.

Over-the-Counter Estriol

As a woman moves into perimenopause, irregular periods signal that estrogen levels are no longer sufficient to stimulate monthly menstruation. Other symptoms of declining estrogen levels can include decreased libido, hot flashes, vaginal dryness, and vaginal atrophy (thinning of the vaginal walls) that may cause intercourse to be painful. Many women find that they are able to safely eliminate these uncomfortable symptoms by using an over-the-counter bioidentical estriol formulation.

For decades, the traditional medical community considered estriol to be of little clinical significance due to its weak estrogenic activity when compared to estrone and estradiol. Current medical research, however, establishes that bioidentical estriol safely reduces symptoms of menopause—such as hot flashes and vaginal dryness—while also positively impacting bone density, heart health, and brain function. In 1993, the *New England Journal of Medicine* reported that bioidentical estriol should be regarded as the treatment of choice for perimenopausal and menopausal women frequently suffering from incontinence and/or recurrent urinary tract infections. In contrast to the placebo group, women using bioidentical estriol cream intravaginally showed a significant decrease in symptoms and a dramatic reduction in recurrent infections.[1]

Unlike its more potent "sister" estrogens (estrone and estradiol) or dangerous synthetic estrogens (such as Premarin), studies validate that bioidentical estriol supports optimum hormone balance without increasing the risk of hormone-dependent cancers of the breast and endometrium. Transdermal (through the skin) administration of bioidentical estriol has been shown to be more effective than oral formulations.

Estriol cream should be applied vaginally and to the forearms. If your symptoms persist after using both over-the-counter progesterone and estriol creams for four to six weeks, over-the-counter strengths are no longer sufficient. You will need to find a physician who will order lab work and analyze your personal hormone-level profile before writing a prescription for exactly the mix and dosage of BHRT your body is crying for.

Your Personal Hormone-Level Profile

Hormone levels can be measured by blood, urine, or saliva tests, based on your physician's preference. A complete and individualized hormone-level profile is needed to provide a rational basis for correcting anything more than the initial downshift in progesterone production. This profile should include measurements of both free, or bioavailable, and total hormones.

When the endocrine system manufactures sex hormones, they are released into the bloodstream bound to carrier proteins. Only a small fraction (1 to 5 percent) of a given amount of a sex hormone breaks loose from the carrier protein in the bloodstream and is free to enter the target tissues. This free or unbound hormone is bioavailable to act on target tissues such as the breast, uterus, brain, colon, bones, heart, arteries, and skin.

In addition to determining bioavailable levels of the sex hormones, a complete hormone profile must include analysis of the other hormones not bound to carrier proteins. These include the thyroid hormones (TSH, T3, T4, and thyroid peroxidase) and the adrenal hormones (cortisol and DHEA sulfate).

Newer, more ultrasensitive blood tests called radioimmune assays (RIA) given an accurate reading of bioavailable and other required hormone levels, thereby providing a complete hormone-level profile in a single test. The table on page 79 indicates the blood work Randy typically orders for our female and male patients.

For a more comprehensive evaluation of overall health status, blood work analysis should also include:

- Comprehensive metabolic profile (CMP): checks blood sugar, electrolytes, kidney and liver function, globulin and albumin levels

Women	Hormones	Men	Hormones
Ovarian	Estradiol Estrone Progesterone Testosterone (free and total)	Testicular	Estradiol Progesterone Testosterone (free and total) Dihydrotestosterone (DHT)
Adrenal	DHEA sulfate Cortisol, 8:00 A.M.*	Adrenal	DHEA sulfate Cortisol, 8:00 A.M.*
Pituitary	Follicle- stimulating hormone (FSH) Luteinizing hormone (LH)	Pituitary	Follicle-stimulating hormone (FSH) Luteinizing hormone (LH)
Thyroid	Thyroid–stimulating hormone (TSH) T3 free T4 free Thyroid peroxidase antibody (TPA)	Thyroid	Thyroid–stimulating hormone (TSH) T3 free T4 free Thyroid peroxidase antibody (TPA)

* If 8:00 A.M. cortisol levels are not in the normal range, other tests will be ordered.

- Lipid profile: measures triglycerides, total cholesterol, and ratio of good (HDL) to bad (LDL) cholesterol
- Markers for cardiovascular disease: C-reactive protein (CRP) and homocysteine
- Vitamin D levels: 25-hydroxy-vitamin D
- Ovarian cancer test (if ovaries are present): Ca-125

Saliva testing accurately measures tissue levels of the bio-available sex hormones, but it cannot measure levels of other important hormones, such as FSH, LH, and the hormones produced by the thyroid gland (TSH, T3, T4, and thyroid peroxidase). To obtain a complete hormone profile, salivary tests must be augmented with finger-stick dried blood spot testing or RIA blood tests.

A urine sample can provide a complete hormone profile if analyzed with gas chromatography coupled with mass spectrometry (GC/MS). This testing modality is used to detect illicit steroid hormone use among athletes, including those participating in the Olympics. However, owing to high equipment and personnel costs associated with the sophisticated equipment and methodology, GC/MS analysis has largely been confined to universities and medical schools.

Your physician will analyze your hormone-level profile to determine which hormones you will need and the amounts to reestablish hormonal equilibrium at a cellular level. Your individualized composite of BHRT will be specially prepared in a compounding pharmacy.

Your Personalized BHRT Prescription

With your lab work in hand, a physician will know exactly which hormones your body is missing. You may need a prescription for a higher concentration of bioidentical progesterone, or you may need bioidentical progesterone plus bioidentical estrogen and/or testosterone.

In the perimenopausal years, women frequently need to augment bioidentical progesterone replacement with bioidentical estrogen and bioidentical testosterone to restore optimum hormone balance. Menopausal women and women who have had a partial or complete hysterectomy will need a full panel of all three sex hormones.

There are three types of estrogen commonly used in BHRT:

estrone (E1), estradiol (E2), and estriol (E3), the weakest of the three. Bioidentical estrogen compounds are prepared in various combinations of these three types of estrogen. Years ago, the most common was Triest, a formulation of 10 percent estrone, 10 percent estradiol, and 80 percent estriol. Because estrone can be converted into very carcinogenic metabolites, most physicians now prefer to prescribe Biest, a formulation of estradiol and estriol only.

This is very important (and is often overlooked by physicians who are inexperienced in prescribing BHRT): Even if the estrogen you are taking is bioidentical, *you always need to take/use bioidentical progesterone* to balance estrogen's ability to stimulate cell growth. Remember, too much cell growth can be a precursor to cancer.

If your hormone profile indicates that a testosterone deficiency has pulled the plug on your well of sexual energy and desire, I have good news. Controlled studies show that bioidentical testosterone replacement restores sexual drive, arousal, and frequency of sexual fantasies in aging women. Restoring youthful testosterone levels in women has been medically proven to improve mood and well-being, and to provide many other health-enhancing benefits, including improved body composition and cardiovascular health.[2] Multiple studies show that restoring testosterone levels to optimum physiologic range may help guard women against breast cancer.[3]

Men and Testosterone

Men may also need lab work to quantify their hormone-level deficits. Though Randy is a board-certified gynecologist, one out of every three patients he treats is a man desperately seeking help for low libido or sexual dysfunction. Many of these men have been told by other physicians that their testosterone levels are normal. Such was the case with 45-year-old Stanford:

> Until three years ago, I took pride in the fact that I could sustain an erection for a half hour or more of intensive sexual activity and intercourse. Now, if I get an erection, I barely make penetration before ejaculating. I went to see a urologist, who tested for low testosterone, but he said my levels were within normal limits. He suggested I practice a male form of Kegel exercises, where I start peeing, then stop, and hold it while I count to three, then pee again. I feel like an idiot standing in the bathroom performing like a start-stop sprinkler, but I would do it all day long if it helped, but it has not. Could that doctor have possibly read my test results wrong?

Randy explained to Stanford that it was possible that his urologist ordered lab work measuring his total testosterone levels, but those results can be deceptive. He repeated Stanford's blood tests and also analyzed the amount of free testosterone circulating within his system. Read on to understand why Stanford's second test yielded very different results.

Free Versus Total Testosterone

Testosterone circulates in the blood in three forms:

1. About 40 percent of testosterone is bound tightly to sexual hormone-binding globulin (SHBG) and is not available to body tissues for action.

2. About 58 percent is weakly bound to another protein called albumin and is available to many tissues for action.

3. About 2 percent circulates freely in the bloodstream.

Low testosterone is best diagnosed from the results of three different blood tests measuring levels of total testosterone, free testosterone, and SHBG. A normal total testosterone reading may not necessarily indicate that a man has normal levels of free testosterone. For example, some men with increased levels of SHBG and low levels of free testosterone may have normal levels of total testosterone. Medical experts agree that free testosterone is the best indicator of a man's testosterone status.

Bioidentical Testosterone Gets You Back in the Saddle Again

Medical studies have proven that bioidentical testosterone helps men reclaim a youthful enthusiasm for sex. Even better, the benefits include:

- Improvement in erectile function
- Increased bone density and minerals
- Increased energy
- Decreased body fat
- Increased muscle strength
- Decreased heart disease

The health benefits of bioidentical testosterone replacement are sometimes overshadowed by its reputation for abuse and concerns about side effects. To set the record straight, let's examine the facts.

I Don't Want to Turn Into "the Hulk"

Phil, a 46-year-old high school history teacher with a slight build, expressed concern about taking testosterone:

> I want to have more energy and my sex drive back, but I just don't know about this idea of my taking testosterone. I have never wanted to be a gym rat, so if I started bulking up like that muscle-bound green Hulk on that old television show, I wouldn't feel like I was in my own body. With all the press about athletes illegally using steroids, isn't that stuff hard to get hold of, anyway?

Testosterone belongs in the chemical family of anabolic steroids. In his book *Resetting the Clock*, Elmer M. Cranton states, "Testosterone has a terrible reputation. We all have images of overdeveloped and overambitious athletes taking illegal steroids on the q.t. to gain an edge, their biceps bulging like melons about ready to pop through the tightly stretched, fat-free flesh of their arms."[4] After a series of scandals and negative publicity in the 1980s (such as Ben Johnson's improved performance in the 1988 Summer Olympics), rules prohibiting anabolic steroid use were strengthened by many sports organizations. Medical research and the media publicized the dangers of unnatural levels of steroid hormones, including sterility, coronary artery disease, liver damage, and brain tumors. In response to the concern about their potential abuse, testosterone and other anabolic steroids were designated as controlled substances by Congress in 1990.

Just as safe bioidentical progesterone is often confused with dangerous synthetic progestin, bioidentical testosterone often gets a bum rap because it is confused with synthetic versions, which are unsafe. The synthetic versions have a different molecular structure than the testosterone produced by the body and are twenty to fifty times more potent than bioidentical testosterone and the testosterone produced by the body.

So will bioidentical testosterone supplementation turn you into a muscle-bound monster with health problems? Not if the dosage is the amount needed to restore optimum levels. The dosage of bioidentical testosterone used to treat low libido and erectile dysfunction is far less than that used—or abused—for sports purposes. Your physician will monitor your testosterone levels to ensure that you get healthy and sexy but are never at risk of becoming "the Hulk."

What About Testosterone Supplementation and Prostate Cancer Risk?

At 52, Patrick was at the zenith of his career as a defense attorney. Divorced for five years, he had been recently dubbed one of Florida's ten most eligible bachelors over 40. But he had problems:

> Last week, I escorted a 34-year-old blonde bombshell to a charity auction. After the event, she invited me back to her place for a drink. Like something out of a movie, she excused herself to go the bathroom and returned buck naked. One look at her gorgeous body should have immediately had me in tripod stance, if you know what I mean. Unfortunately, my willie popped to attention for a moment or two, then wilted away. I was humiliated. I lied that I was on some new medication with sexual side effects, but I'm not. It's been over a year since I have been able to keep it up long enough to have sex.
>
> My best friend, Jack, said you helped him get back into and up for sex with testosterone shots. I don't want to continue to

feel like a eunuch, but my internist told me that testosterone supplementation would increase my risk of prostate cancer. Is that true?

Men are rightly fearful of prostate cancer, now the second highest killer cancer in males, and like Patrick, this sometimes makes them hesitant to embrace testosterone replacement. Chapter 2 blew away the myth that high testosterone levels cause prostate cancer. Contrary to the beliefs of many physicians, medical evidence validates that *low* testosterone levels increase prostate cancer risk. According to Abraham Morgentaler, a Harvard Medical School professor and author of *Testosterone for Life*, "The long-standing fear about testosterone replacement and prostate cancer has little scientific support. Treatment with testosterone does not increase the risk of prostate cancer, even among men who are already at high risk for it."[5] In fact, testosterone can be safely given to men with prostate cancer if properly monitored.

Bioidentical testosterone treatments are available in several forms, including lozenges, sublingual drops, gels, patches, injections, and slow-release testosterone pellets inserted under the skin, usually in the buttocks. The pill form of bioidentical testosterone is strongly discouraged due to liver toxicity and poor absorption.

Men on bioidentical testosterone replacement therapy should be monitored by their physician to ensure that testosterone levels remain within the normal range. A digital rectal examination (DRE) should be performed and prostate-specific antigen (PSA) checked in all men before initiating treatment. These tests should be repeated at approximately three to six months, and

then biannually in men over 40 years of age. The physician prescribing testosterone replacement should also evaluate changes in
clinical symptoms and assess for other concerns, such as acne and
increase in breast size and tenderness.

*Men on any form of testosterone should also be on a 5-alpha reductase
enzyme blocker* (such as bioidentical progesterone cream), because
this decreases the conversion of testosterone to one of its metabolites, dihydrotestosterone (DHT), as well as an aromatase
enzyme blocker (such as the herb chrysin or the hormone melatonin) to decrease the conversion of testosterone to the estrogens
estradiol and estrone. DHT and estrogen are bad for the prostate
and contribute to male pattern baldness as well as weight gain.

If men are on testosterone intramuscular injections, Randy
recommends the prescription-strength blockers finasteride for
5-alpha reductase and anastrazole for aromatase. These prevent
the buildup of DHT and estrogen and are stronger than progesterone, chrysin, and melatonin.

DHEA Supplementation for Women and Men

DHEA has been heralded as the antiaging hormone for women
and men. Clinical studies have found that supplementing to sustain optimum DHEA levels can contribute to cardiovascular
health, protect against deterioration of mental functioning and
depression, prevent osteoporosis, and help the immune system
fight disease. Other benefits include improved libido and enhanced sexual performance. If your personal hormone-level profile shows that cortisol and/or DHEA levels are elevated or
depressed, your doctor will know that stress is a factor in your
increasingly sexless life.

Because DHEA can be converted to testosterone and estrogen, its supplementation is not quite as simple as quantifying the deficiency and replacing what is missing. DHEA supplementation, whether prescription or over the counter, should always be monitored by lab work. Women and men should consider repeating a hormone-level profile three to six weeks after beginning DHEA therapy to determine optimal dosing, then every three months while on the regimen.

Women who have been diagnosed with an estrogen-dependent cancer should consider taking 7-keto DHEA, which will not convert to estrogen or testosterone, or should work closely with a physician to evaluate DHEA's effect on estrogen levels. If DHEA were to elevate estrogen levels too much, this could theoretically increase the risk of cancer recurrence.

Similarly, men with prostate cancer or prostate disease should either take 7-keto DHEA or avoid DHEA altogether. Therefore, men should have a PSA and a DRE before initiating DHEA therapy to rule out existing prostate disease. Medical evidence indicates that maintaining youthful DHEA levels may protect against prostate cancer.

The Difference Between a Compounding Pharmacy and Your Corner Drugstore

Compounding pharmacies are different from your neighborhood drugstore. Whereas drugstores dispense ready-made drugs in preset dosages, compounding pharmacies customize individual prescriptions. Prescriptions can vary in dosage strength, choices of custom fillers (for example, lactose-free), and options of delivery, including creams, sublingual (under the tongue) drops, tablets, capsules, liquids, lozenges, patches, pellets, and in-jections. Depending on what hormone formulations you need and your own doctor's personal approach to BHRT, you might fill a prescription at either a corner drugstore or a compounding pharmacy.

Compounding pharmacists utilize ingredients approved by the U.S. Pharmacopeia (USP) as pure and micronized, which means that the product is a fine grade that will be well absorbed into your system, resulting in less waste being processed through the digestive system. Bioidentical hormones from a compound-ing pharmacy can be prescribed as long-acting or sustained re-lease. This helps the body have a more balanced hormone level instead of the highs and lows that can come with some pharma-ceutically manufactured products.

Pharmaceutical Industry Champions of BHRT

Some forward-thinking pharmaceutical companies have begun to manufacture proprietary bioidentical hormone products ap-proved by the FDA. While these specialty biopharmaceutical companies cannot patent the bioidentical hormone molecule, they can patent its delivery mechanism or dosage form. These products are far superior options to synthetic HRT, but their limitation is that the concentration of bioidentical hormone they contain cannot be titrated (increased or decreased) based on individual response. For those physicians and patients who may have a higher comfort level with a standardized manufactured product, however, these bioidentical products are very good op-tions. Prescriptions for these products can be filled at your neigh-borhood drugstore.

Bioidentical Estradiol	Bioidentical Progesterone	Bioidentical Testosterone
Divigel	Prochieve	AndroGel
Estrasorb	Prometrium	Testopel
EstroGel		
Evamist		
Estrace		

Now don't grab hold of your first prescription for BHRT too tightly. The mix of bioidentical hormones you need right now to recharge your sexual battery is going to change as you age.

6

BHRT Is Not Everyone's Sexual Saving Grace

After reading the last chapter, you may be chomping at the bit to get a prescription for BHRT to start rejuvenating your sex life from the inside out. Hold off from rushing to call your doctor until after you have read this chapter. While BHRT is an excellent option for some people seeking a natural and medically proven approach to sexual restoration, it is not a panacea for everyone. Hurdles associated with access, cost, controversial approaches, and a battle of international scope may get in your way.

Hurdle 1: Finding a Doctor Who Will Prescribe BHRT

Wondering why your doctor hasn't already told you about BHRT? Excellent question with a simple answer. Many physicians have only recently begun to consider bioidentical hormone replacement as a viable treatment.

Physicians have been trained in medical school to prescribe

synthetic hormones. Once out of medical school, they rely on education from continuing medical education (CME) programs and pharmaceutical representatives to keep them abreast of new research. Unfortunately, physician scientists researching bioidentical hormones (for example, Joel Hargrove at Vanderbilt University Medical School in Nashville, Tennessee; Helene Leonetti at St. Luke's Medical Center in Bethlehem, Pennsylvania; Kenna Stephenson at the University of Texas in Tyler) do not have a budget for mass marketing or a sales force to facilitate the distribution of their research findings to physician peers across the country.

BHRT owes its increasing popularity to celebrities, including Oprah Winfrey, Suzanne Somers, and Robin McGraw, who have gotten the word out on a national scale. By broadcasting their personal testimonies on television programs and in books and magazines, these high-profile women have motivated millions of women to learn more about BHRT. They have also become a thorn in the side of conventional physicians. The average woman is researching BHRT on the Internet and in articles and books before making an appointment with her doctor. These informed health care consumers are forcing doctors to play catch-up.

If you are interested in finding a doctor who is experienced in treating low libido and sexual dysfunction with BHRT, you may have to cast a wide net. While more and more doctors are attending CME programs to learn about this emerging field, the number of BHRT specialists in the United States is not yet sufficient to meet an ever-increasing demand. "How do I find a doctor who can prescribe BHRT?" continues to be the number one question received on our Web site, www.hormonewell.com.

In addition to issues associated with acceptance and access, the field of bioidentical hormone replacement medicine is sometimes compromised by a lack of medical integrity. Some more entrepreneurial physicians witnessing the increasing consumer demand for BHRT are entering this field from a marketing, rather than a medical, perspective. They read a book or attend an afternoon seminar, then add bioidentical hormone replacement to their line of services. This can be dangerous. The complexities of analyzing hormone deficiencies and monitoring physiologic levels requires a level of competency that can take years to develop. You may need help to decipher credible medical professionals from noncredible medical marketers.

If you want to find a physician you can trust as a BHRT medical expert, I suggest you begin your search by asking your local compounding pharmacist. He or she will know which doctors in your area are writing prescriptions for BHRT. If you are unsure how to locate a compounding pharmacy, Appendix B provides you with the contact information for two national associations that can help you: the International Association of Compounding Pharmacists (IACP) and the Professional Compounding Centers of America (PCCA).

When you meet your new BHRT specialist for the first time, ask him or her the following questions:

1. How long have you been using BHRT to treat patients with low libido, sexual dysfunction, and other symptoms of hormone imbalance?

2. Where and with whom did you train? (*Note:* Do an Internet search and check out the faculty and program.)

3. What is your approach to monitoring hormone levels both short and long term?

4. Understanding patient privacy concerns, do you have two or

three patients who would be willing to share their experience
with me?

Hurdle 2: The Out-of-Pocket Expense

LaDonna, a 47-year-old perimenopausal woman, sent us this
e-mail:

> For two years, I sweated, screamed, suffered irregular periods,
> and ditched my sex life. Then I saw a television program on bio-
> identical hormones and felt as if I had been handed a get-out-
> of-jail-free card. The problem is that I soon discovered that
> these hormones are definitely not free. I spoke to three different
> doctors' offices and was told that my initial evaluation could
> cost close to one thousand dollars. Then I would have to pay out
> of pocket each month for my personalized prescription of
> BHRT. I can't afford those fees. It's back to suffering and no sex
> for me.

Some physicians specializing in BHRT do accept insurance,
but many do not. Out-of-pocket costs will vary by provider and
can range from hundreds to thousands of dollars. Some doctors
will provide you with an invoice that you can submit directly to
your insurance provider.

The Hotze Health & Wellness Center in Houston, Texas,
is nationally recognized as a center of excellence in using bioidentical hormones to treat hypothyroidism, adrenal fatigue, and
hormone imbalances. According to its Web site, www.hotzehwc
.com, the cost of its personalized hormone replacement program
can range from $1,100 to $3,900.[1] Similarly, BodyLogicMD, a

national network of physicians trained in BHRT, cites the following costs on its Web site, www.bodylogicmd.com:

- $275–$395 for initial visit
- $450–$595 for initial lab work
- $275 for follow-up visits occurring at month three and then every six months thereafter
- $250 for follow-up lab work; may vary depending on BHRT regimen
- $100 for average monthly cost of BHRT and recommended supplements.[2]

To calculate BodyLogic's approximate cost for the first year, I assumed two follow-up visits requiring two series of follow-up lab work, bringing the total cost to $3,240.

These out-of-pocket costs are beyond the range of most people, causing BHRT to be categorized as an elective luxury rather than a health care necessity. And the sad news is that this gap can be expected to widen unless significant changes occur in health care and insurance legislation at the national level.

Hurdle 3: Sorting Through Controversial Approaches

If you think that BHRT could be the sexual jump-start you have been waiting for, you need to be aware that some approaches are more controversial than others. Consider the Wiley Protocol advocated by Suzanne Somers in *Ageless*.

The Wiley Protocol

Elena sat in the front row nodding her head through most of my luncheon lecture. When the floor was opened for questions, her hand was the first to shoot up.

> I am 58 years old and have been out of menopause for five years now. I love the idea that I might once again be energetic, excited, and sexually vital, but I don't want to trick my body into thinking I am so young that I start having periods again. Is that necessary?

I told Elena that this drastic method of hormone replacement therapy is indeed not necessary or even recommended. The Wiley Protocol was first devised by T. S. Wiley, author of *Lights Out: Sleep, Sugar and Survival* and *Sex, Lies and Menopause*. The protocol claims to relieve the symptoms of menopause, but it is also promoted as an approach to increasing overall health. It involves using rhythmic doses of hormones to re-create the premenopausal monthly cycle—that is, it uses high dosages of bioidentical hormones to force a menopausal woman to have periods.

While Randy and I applaud Ms. Somers for her willingness to use her celebrity status to raise awareness about BHRT, we have grave concerns about this protocol. The Wiley Protocol uses high nonphysiologic dosages of hormones, which many medical experts agree could be dangerous. Furthermore, Wiley's lack of any formal medical education or training is an issue. Finally, significant side effects have been reported by women on this protocol. BHRT should not necessarily cause menopausal women to continue to menstruate. We recommend a much more conservative BHRT approach.

Human Growth Hormone

Santo, who is 52, came to his appointment with Randy carrying a file folder full of Internet advertisements for human growth hormone (HGH):

> Dr. Randolph, I saw this Internet ad saying that this human growth hormone spray would help me grow younger almost overnight. I was about to order a six-month supply because it was on sale from $400 to $300, but my girlfriend insisted I come to see you first to make sure I wouldn't be throwing my money away. She also wants me to find out if this stuff is safe. Is it?

Bioidentical supplementation of HGH is under scrutiny as an all-purpose tonic. HGH is secreted by the pituitary gland and contributes to muscle growth, tissue repair, physical and mental health, bone strength, energy, metabolism, and sexual appetite. Production peaks in adolescence, then declines about 14 percent every ten years.

Referred to as the fountain-of-youth hormone, HGH is said to enhance virility and potency in men and promote multiple orgasms in women. Demand for HGH has soared in recent years, with an increasing number of HGH products being sold over the Internet, but let the buyer beware. According to physicians at the Mayo Clinic, taking HGH can cause a number of side effects,[3] including:

- Swelling in the arms and legs
- Arthritis-like symptoms
- Carpal tunnel symptoms

- Headaches
- Bloating
- Muscle pain
- Diabetes
- Abnormal growth of bones and internal organs
- Hardening of the arteries
- High blood pressure

Some evidence shows that side effects of HGH treatments may be more likely in older adults. Because the studies of healthy adults taking HGH have been short term, it is not known whether these side effects could eventually dissipate or become worse. For instance, though HGH produced arthritis-like symptoms, it isn't clear if this would progress into arthritis. When it comes to using HGH to treat low libido and/or sexual dysfunction, our medical opinion is that the jury is still out.

Hurdle 4: Pharmaceutical Companies Are Fighting BHRT

From pharmaceutical manufacturer Wyeth's perspective, the increasing consumer interest in BHRT is not necessarily a good development. When women opt out of synthetic hormone drugs and instead ask their physicians for BHRT, millions of dollars of pharmaceutical company revenue is at stake. Not surprisingly, in 2008, Wyeth threw down the gauntlet. A battle that had been simmering for decades began to boil in the open.

In January 2008, the FDA announced that it would halt the compounding of hormones that contained estriol. This announcement was made in a press conference and in a series of letters sent to seven compounding pharmacies. The enforcement actions against estriol were requested in a citizen petition filed in 2005 by Wyeth.[4]

The FDA's announcement sparked a grassroots initiative of momentous proportions. In response to the outpouring of protest from thousands of women across the United States whose right to use estriol could be taken away, members of the House of Representatives stepped up and introduced a bipartisan resolution that reads as follows: "Expressing the sense of Congress that the Food and Drug Administration's (FDA) new policy restricting women's access to medications containing estriol does not serve the public interest." The estriol resolution was introduced by Mike Ross (D-Ark.), Jo Ann Emerson (R-Mo.), Tammy Baldwin (D-Wis.), Michael Burgess (R-Texas), John Carter (R-Texas), Sam Farr (D-Calif.), and Gabrielle Giffords (D-Ariz.). Score one for BHRT, strike one for Wyeth.

In January 2009, as a direct rebuttal to two *Oprah* television segments on BHRT, the medical journal *OBG Management* published the cover story "Bio-identical Hormones: What You (and Your Patient) Need to Know." The tagline on the cover read: "Here's the skinny on compounded 'bio-identical' hormone therapy—popular among women but absolutely data-free."[5] The article noted that the American College of Obstetricians and Gynecologists (ACOG), the North American Menopause Society (NAMS), and the Endocrine Society had all issued statements noting the lack of safety data on compounded bioidentical hormones; however, no studies or medical evidence were cited to support the premise that BHRT is unsafe.

Joann V. Pinkerton was the author of this article. A sidebar noted that Pinkerton is a paid consultant for Wyeth and other pharmaceutical companies. Across this country and around the globe, medical scientists researching BHRT rose up in arms calling for a comprehensive and *unbiased review* of all the medical literature on BHRT.

There is a need for a government-funded large randomized clinical trial comparing BHRT to synthetic HRT. The big question is: Who will fund this study? The National Institutes of Health (NHI) and Wyeth funded the Women's Health Initiative study. Hopefully, the government will once again step up to the plate, this time without a pharmaceutical partner as sponsor, and allow indisputable scientific data to settle this battle once and for all.

BHRT may not be right for you if you can't find a doctor, afford the therapy, or feel comfortable going against the tide of mainstream medicine. Don't worry. You are not condemned to sink deeper into a sexual stupor because of untreated hormone deficiencies. BHRT is only one natural option for restoring hormone balance. Read on to find out about three others.

Part Three:

Back in the Groove:
Three Steps That Naturally Boost
and Balance Hormone Levels

If you want to rejuvenate your sex life but are not sure whether BHRT is for you, or if you are currently taking bioidentical hormones but want to fan your sexual flames even more, our three-step plan is great. This integrative approach to rejuvenating sexuality is spawned from a unique synergy among specific foods (Chapter 7), natural supplements (Chapter 8), and lifestyle choices (Chapter 9). It is safe, simple, low cost, and doesn't require a prescription.

Think of our three steps to sexual rejuvenation as three phases in building a house. Step 1 (diet) lays the foundation; step 2 (natural supplements) puts up the walls and the roof; and step 3 (lifestyle choices) turns on the electricity, moves in the furniture, and puts sheets on the bed. Diet is the foundation for sexual restoration, but natural supplements, including plant-based or phytohormones, will be needed to get the new sexual you up and going. If you want to experience maximum sexual voltage, you'll learn how to flip that switch with exercise, stress management, and a good night's sleep. Fully embrace all three steps and we guarantee you will say a permanent good-bye to your fading libido, flagging energy, and flabby body and a happy hello to your new hormone-sexy life.

7

Step 1:
Eat Foods to Fuel Your Sexual Fire

If your libido has gone down the tubes because of hormone imbalance, it's time for you to change your diet. A consistent diet of sexy-healthy foods will not only improve your sexuality, it will make you fitter, healthier, and raring to go. Ditch the Viagra or the stiletto heels—a trip to the grocery store is your first step toward the best sex of your life.

Sexy-Healthy Eating

When Caleb and Latisha walked into my consultation room, I was immediately struck by the difference in their physiques. Whereas six-foot-two Caleb was so thin his elbows and knees protruded sharply through his flannel shirt and woolen pants, five-foot-one Latisha resembled a Rubenesque cherub swabbed in yards of crimson and black silk. As if reading my thoughts, Latisha opened our conversation:

Don't we look like Mutt and Jeff? But I tell you, that never did matter much to us. I was only sixteen the first time I laid eyes on this man, and I knew then and there that he would be the one kissing me in front of the altar even if I had to stand on an orange crate to reach his lips. Now, forty years later, I am still crazy about him. The problem is that we have stopped being crazy for each other in a sexual way. My mother used to say, "The minute you stop feeling frisky in the bedroom is the first minute of your funeral," so you can see why I want to turn this around.

I think we don't have sex because I have gotten so fat that my "down there" is literally suffocating. Caleb claims that he is the one with the problem. He tells me, "My love spirit is strong, but my manhood is weak." We are here because I want an expert opinion on who is right. If it is me, I want a diet pill. If it is Caleb, he can take the medicine Senator Dole talked about on television. What do you think?

"I think you are both right," I told them. "But rather than give you prescriptions, I am going to send you out the door with a grocery list and some recipes."

Wondering how I knew the right diet would recharge Latisha and Caleb's sexual batteries? Let me explain.

At 56 years old, age-related testosterone-level decline was undoubtedly a concern for both. Weight was another shared issue, though with different consequences. Though menopausal, Latisha was suffering from body fat–induced estrogen dominance. In contrast, Caleb's lack of body fat was causing his testosterone levels to lag. Both needed a diet designed to balance their hormones and support favorable weight management.

Three things must be considered. The first is that while

women and men will undoubtedly have very different hormone deficiencies, both sexes will benefit from a diet rich in foods that balance estrogen levels and boost testosterone production. Latisha and Caleb, for instance, used the same recipes and sat down to the same meals.

The second is that while the sexy-healthy food plan promotes weight loss and a healthier body mass composition, it is not a calorie-counting program. My experience has been that as the body moves back into a state of hormone balance, food cravings subside and you are more prone to eat food as fuel. This means you relearn to eat based on feelings of hunger and fullness. Counting calories is synonymous with dieting. We recommend a plan that is much more than a temporary approach to weight loss; it is a lifetime approach to eating your way toward better sex.

The third is that while diet is the foundation of hormone health, diet alone is probably not your answer. To restore youthful sexual function without bioidentical hormone replacement, you will need the help of natural supplements and the willingness to commit to hormone healthy-sexy lifestyle choices. These essential components will be described in Chapters 8 and 9.

With those caveats in mind, let's start your grocery list.

Choose Organic When Possible

When you go to the grocery store or produce market, buy organic foods when possible and within your budget. The term *organic food* is usually taken to mean a food that has been produced without artificial fertilizers and has not been subject to treatment with growth hormones, synthetic pesticides, or any antibiotics. In 2002, a startling 47 percent of the produce sampled by the

U.S. Department of Agriculture (USDA) had detectable pesticide residues.

New data indicates that eating hormone-treated meat may increase estrogen levels hundreds of times over what the body naturally produces. It's disputed at this point just how much synthetic hormone ends up on the dinner plate. Beef cows in the United States are implanted with multiple synthetic hormones, including estradiol, to make them put on weight. There is no withdrawal period for these implants, which are in the cows at the time of slaughter. They're outlawed in Europe and not used in developing countries, but they are routinely implanted in cows in North America, Australia, New Zealand, and Argentina. North America has the highest rate of breast and prostate cancers in the world. The number of cases of breast cancer in Australia and New Zealand alone almost equals the number for all of Central America, including Mexico.[1] As you learned in Chapter 3, these xenoestrogens can upset hormone balance and have a toxic effect on your health.

Eat to Support Estrogen Balance

Estrogen balance is essential for you to feel and act sexy. Before you learn about how to eat to support estrogen balance, let's review the sexual ramification of too much or too little estrogen.

Estrogen dominance causes you to lose your libido, gain weight, and feel awful all over. Estrogen's propensity to promote cell growth is left unopposed. And don't forget that estrogen dominance is not just a woman's affliction. Men carrying around extra body fat can also have their sex drive sabotaged by this underlying condition.

In a different way, estrogen deficiency compromises sexual performance and pleasure. Perimenopausal women, menopausal women, and women who have had a partial or complete hysterectomy can't produce enough estrogen to lubricate vaginally. Vaginal walls also weaken, resulting in painful intercourse.

At a cellular level, estrogen equilibrium is a very sensitive teeter-totter. The good news is that one of the most effective mechanisms for balancing your inner estrogen teeter-totter is not only safe, it is also quite tasty. It requires that you eat more phytoestrogens.

Foods Rich in Phytoestrogens

Phytoestrogen literally means "plant estrogen"; however, this term is something of a misnomer. The National Cancer Institute currently defines phytoestrogens as "estrogen-like substances found in some plants and plant products." According to nurse practitioner Marcelle Pick, cofounder of Women to Women, "Phytoestrogens have a chemical structure that allows them to temporarily and weakly bind to the body's estrogen receptors, potentially blocking excess estrogen or quieting the system's need for more estrogen.[2] That is, if you are estrogen dominant, phytoestrogens will temporarily bind to your estrogen receptors, thereby reducing estrogen activity at a cellular level. Conversely, if you are estrogen deficient, phytoestrogens will jump in to make up for some of the insufficiency.

Each time I explain how phytoestrogens function within the body, I am reminded of this childhood joke:

It is the 1960s and three little boys are debating the most wondrous invention of their time.

"I think it is the airplane," says the first little boy. "It can go up in the sky and carry hundreds of people all over the world to see their grandparents."

"Naw," says the second little boy. "That ain't it. I think the most wondrous invention is the spaceship. It can take men up in the sky, where they eat dried-up pieces of food before walking on the moon."

"I think you are both wrong," the third little boy confidently asserts. "The most wondrous invention of all time is the thermos."

"The thermos?" the first two little boys chorus in disbelief. "Why in the world would you say the thermos?"

"Because it can keep hot things hot and cold things cold. Think about it. . . . How does it know?"

The biochemical term for the "how-does-it-know" phenomenon of phytoestrogens is *selective estrogen receptor modulators*, or SERMs. Because of their unique modulating response, foods and supplements containing phytoestrogens do not promote estrogen dominance nor do they in any way contribute to unbalanced cell growth that can increase your risk of cancer.

In addition to their ability to suppress menopausal discomforts in women—particularly vasomotor symptoms like hot flashes and night sweats—numerous studies have shown that some phytoestrogens may have significant cancer-fighting capabilities, particularly in the colon, uterus, and breast.[3] In 1999, the FDA authorized the use of food-label health claims connecting increased phytoestrogen consumption with reduced risk of coronary heart disease. One study of more than four hundred women demonstrated that phytoestrogens protect against arterial degeneration and atherosclerosis, particularly in older women.

Some of the richest phytoestrogen-containing foods are soy

products, including soybeans, soy milk, tofu, tempeh, textured vegetable protein, roasted soybeans, miso, and edamame. Did you know that the Japanese do not have a word for hot flash? Because the Japanese diet is rich in phytoestrogens, Japanese women may experience less hot flashes than American women.

Lignans are another exemplary phytoestrogenic food group. Lignans are present in a wide variety of plant foods, including seeds (flax, flaxseed oil, pumpkin, sunflower, poppy), whole grains (rye, oats, barley), bran (wheat, oat, rye), fruits (particularly berries), and some vegetables. Flaxseed is by far the richest dietary source of plant lignans.

Foods That Promote Healthy Estrogen Metabolism and Elimination

In addition to eating a diet rich in phytoestrogens, eating more of the following foods can positively impact how your body metabolizes and eliminates estrogen:

- **Cruciferous vegetables:** Cruciferous vegetables include broccoli, asparagus, cauliflower, spinach, Brussels sprouts, celery, beet root, kale, cabbage, parsley root, radishes, turnips, collards, and mustard greens. Estrogen can be metabolized in the body to be "good" or "bad." Cruciferous vegetables contain a phytonutrient called indole-3-carbinol (I3C). I3C has been shown to act as a catalyst to pull estradiol down a benign pathway to 2-hydroxyestrone, thus decreasing levels of the carcinogenic 16-alpha-hydroxyestrone. Simply stated, cruciferous vegetables can help decrease the body's load of unhealthy estrogens and reduce an overall unhealthy condition of estrogen dominance. Additionally, studies have shown that a high intake of cruciferous vegetables offers protection from developing breast cancer.

  Note: Limit your intake of raw cruciferous vegetables because they contain thyroid inhibitors knows as goitrogens. To make sure that your diet doesn't stimulate a case of pseudohypothyroidism, lightly steam, blanch, or stir-fry cruciferous vegetables.

- **Citrus fruits:** D-limonene, found in the oils of citrus fruits, has been shown to promote detoxification of estrogen. Common citrus fruits include oranges, grapefruits, tangerines, lemons, limes, and tangelos. When male and female lab mice were given an extract of D-limonene, research showed that they lost weight.

- **Insoluble fiber:** Insoluble fiber binds to extra estrogen in the digestive tract. This extra estrogen is later eliminated through the bowel. Sources of insoluble fiber include whole grains, whole-wheat breads, barley, couscous, brown rice, whole-grain breakfast cereals, wheat bran, seeds, carrots, cucumbers, zucchini, celery, and tomatoes.

Foods That Boost Testosterone

Testosterone is the hormone most known for its sexual-stimulating capacity. If you are a man over 40, your sex drive and performance deteriorate in lockstep with declining testosterone levels. Women also know that their ebbing testosterone production can zap their desire. Women who have had a partial or complete hysterectomy immediately stop producing testosterone. The good news is that you can begin to bolster lagging testosterone levels by increasing your intake of foods high in zinc, essential fatty acids, and vitamin A.

- **Zinc:** Who knew that eating liver could make you a better lover? The reason: Liver is loaded with zinc. Zinc is necessary to maintain optimum levels of testosterone. Inadequate zinc levels prevent the pituitary gland from releasing luteinizing and follicle-stimulating hormones (LH and

FSH), which promote testosterone production. Zinc also inhibits the aromatase enzyme that converts testosterone into excess estrogen.

In addition to its positive impact on testosterone levels, zinc has been proven to help the body produce healthier sperm by increasing sperm count and motility. Frequent ejaculation can use up zinc, since it is present in male ejaculate. Consequently, sexually active men should increase their intake of zinc. A USDA study found that semen volume dropped 30 percent when zinc intake was low. Research published in the *Annals of Nutritional Metabolism* found that males who consumed low amounts of zinc exhibited decreased semen volume and serum testosterone concentration.[4]

Zinc deficiency predisposes the prostate to infection (prostatitis), which may lead to enlargement of the prostate gland (prostatic hypertrophy).

Food sources rich in zinc include oysters and other mollusks, beef, liver, poultry, shrimp and crab, nuts and seeds, whole grains, tofu, peanuts and peanut butter, lentils, yogurt, and milk. *Note:* Excessive sugar intake uses up the body's supply of zinc.

- **Essential fatty acid (EFA):** Studies have shown that dietary fat has a direct relationship with testosterone production. An increase in certain types of dietary fat seems to bring on an increase in testosterone levels. And a decrease in dietary fat is usually accompanied by a decrease in free testosterone levels. However, you need to eat the right kind of fats to increase your intake of EFAs.

    EFAs are unsaturated fats that are necessary for thousands of biological functions throughout the body. There are two families of EFAs: omega-3 and omega-6. EFA deficiency is common in the United States, particularly omega-3 deficiency. Because EFAs cannot be manufactured by the body, you must get them from the foods you eat. Omega-3 fatty acids not only help increase testosterone production, they also help decrease SHBG (sex hormone-binding globulin) levels, so there is less SHBG to "tie up" available testosterone. In addition, foods high in omega-3 fatty acids make your nervous system function better to improve libido, sexual stamina, and orgasm potential.

Omega-3 fatty acids aid in the prevention of muscle breakdown, help to increase your HDL level (good cholesterol), and support overall hormone balance. Finally, omega-3 fatty acids support emotional well-being and effective brain function. As Clare Vukich, holistic nutritionist, said to me, "A heightened sexual experience can be more readily enjoyed with the care and proper nutrition provided to our most important sex organ . . . the one between our ears!"

Just as with hormones, balance between omega-3 and omega-6 fatty acids is essential. When the ratio between omega-3 and omega-6 fatty acids is optimum, health is supported. Good dietary sources of omega-6 fatty acids can be found in cereals, eggs, poultry, whole-grain breads, and refined vegetable and seed oils (corn, safflower, etc.). Unfortunately, most Americans consume an overabundance of partially refined oils because they are often "hidden" in highly processed, packaged convenience fast foods such as cookies, fried foods, chips, and candy bars. Overconsumption of omega-6 fatty acids promotes inflammation, which can lead to heart disease, type 2 diabetes, arthritis, and rapid aging. The typical American diet tends to contain fourteen to twenty-five times more omega-6 fatty acids than omega-3 fatty acids, and many researchers believe this imbalance is a significant factor in the rising rate of inflammatory disorders in the United States. A healthy diet should consist of roughly two to four times more omega-6 fatty acids than omega-3 fatty acids.[5]

EFA food sources include flaxseed oil, flaxseeds, flaxseed meal, hempseed oil, hempseeds, walnuts, pumpkin seeds, olive oil (extra-virgin or virgin), olives, avocados, almonds, peanuts, sesame oil, pecans, pistachio nuts, cashews, hazelnuts, macadamia nuts, Brazil nuts, sesame seeds, some dark leafy green vegetables (kale, spinach, purslane, mustard greens, collards, etc.), canola oil (cold-pressed and unrefined), soybean oil, wheat germ oil, and oily fish (salmon, mackerel, sardines, anchovies, albacore tuna).

- **Vitamin A:** Vitamin A is necessary for the utilization of protein and the production of testosterone. Abundant animal research correlates vitamin A with testosterone production. An experiment with male rats found that a deficiency in vitamin A causes decreased production of testosterone and testicular atrophy.[6] Another study found that rats with a vitamin A deficiency were 40 percent more likely to develop prostate cancer.[7] The best food sources for vitamin A are liver, egg yolks, full-fat milk, and cod liver oil.

Restore the Sizzle:
What Is Good for Your Heart Is Good for Your Sex Life

Geniva, 49 years old, nervously twisted a tissue before speaking up:

> I just go through the motions, you see. Roosevelt has always been very attentive. In fact, even if he has an orgasm, he doesn't feel sexually satisfied unless I come, too. He doesn't mind stimulating me with his hand or with oral sex. The problem is that in the last few years, I think it would be easier to solve world hunger than for me to climax. I just don't feel things down there like I used to. Can you get the doctor to write me a prescription to help?

"Geniva," I responded, "based on the response of hundreds of women and men who come in here with the same problem, I don't think you will require any medication. You can boost blood flow and restore genital response with a few simple diet changes and increased exercise."

Poor circulation doesn't only cause chilly hands and feet; it decreases sexual sensation and pleasure. No matter how much love you might have in your heart, if your heart is not strongly pumping blood throughout your body including your genital area, your orgasms will be ho-hum if they happen at all. To help your genitals reclaim their sexual sizzle, here are my recommendations for four circulation-stimulating food groups:

1. **Foods rich in L-arginine improve vaginal response and penile performance.** L-arginine is the amino acid that the body uses to create nitric oxide. When you are sexually aroused, your genitals release nitric oxide, which causes blood vessels to expand, engorging the penis or clitoris. If your body is deficient in L-arginine, its supply of nitric oxide will be diminished, and sexual stamina and sensations of pleasure will be weakened. To pump up sexual performance, add more L-arginine-rich foods to your diet. Favorites include nuts and seeds (peanuts, almonds, walnuts, hazelnuts, Brazil nuts, cashews, pecans, pistachio nuts, flaxseeds, and sunflower seeds), granola, oatmeal, canned tuna, salmon, cod, halibut, shrimp, poultry, dried beans, chickpeas, garlic, eggs, green vegetables, and—yippee—dark chocolate.

2. **Antioxidant-loaded vegetables, fruits, and teas (and wine, coffee, and chocolate in moderation) improve circulation to equal better sex.** Oxidants, or free radicals, are molecules within your body that have been damaged by age, stress, and environmental toxins, which cause them to lose an electron. These electron-dispossessed molecules multiply rapidly and damage

other cells. If unstopped, the result of their oxidative rampage may include increased risk of heart disease and cancer, skin damage, wrinkle formation, and accelerated sexual aging.

Antioxidants stop the oxidative damage by replacing the molecule's missing electron, thereby returning the molecule to its original healthy function within your body's cellular society. Antioxidant-rich foods most noted for their sexual-enhancing properties include citrus fruits (oranges, grapefruits, tangelos, tangerines), cruciferous vegetables (broccoli, cauliflower, green leafy vegetables, Brussels sprouts), tomatoes, beets, bell peppers, berries, and red grapes.

Dark chocolate (the higher the cocoa content the better), red wine, black tea, and black coffee all contain the antioxidant polyphenol. Studies have shown that the phenolic constituents, particularly resveratrol and flavonoids, improve blood flow and inhibit the formation of plaque in the arteries. With these antioxidant foods, however, less is definitely more. Consuming more than one cup of caffeinated coffee or tea, one glass of red wine, or one small cube of dark chocolate can respectively tax your adrenals, put you to sleep, or worsen an underlying condition of estrogen dominance. Wine and chocolate can also contribute to weight gain.

3. **Healthy fats and good cholesterol promote production and balance of the sex hormones.** You learned in Chapter 1 that cholesterol is a biochemical building block for all the sex hormones. You can get cholesterol in two ways: Your body makes some cholesterol, and the rest comes from animal products you eat such as meat, poultry, fish, eggs, butter, cheese, and whole and 2 percent milk. Cholesterol is not found in foods from plants.

The medical term for "good" cholesterol is high-density lipoprotein (HDL). HDL carries cholesterol away from your arteries and takes it to your liver, where it's removed from your body. High levels of HDL can protect you from heart attack and stroke and promote sexual health. The medical term for "bad" cholesterol is low-density lipoprotein (LDL). High levels of LDL can clog your arteries, decrease libido and sexual performance, and increase your risk of heart attack and stroke.

Foods high in soluble fiber (such as oatmeal, oat bran, kidney beans, apples, pears, psyllium, barley, and prunes) contain compounds such as hemicellulose, pectins, and lignans that bind to cholesterol in the gut, preventing its absorption. Omega-3 fatty acids, particularly those found in oily cold-water fish, walnuts, flaxseeds, and olive oil, help to reduce blood viscosity and clean the system of cholesterol and fat deposits. These foods also contain a potent mix of antioxidants that can lower LDL but leave HDL untouched.

4. **Cayenne, ginger, and garlic turn up the heat.** Few foods get the blood pumping faster than cayenne, or red pepper. Ginger can also improve circulation. Garlic has been proven to prevent accumulation of plaque in the arteries, thereby improving blood flow.

    You can use cayenne, ginger, and garlic to spice up foods when cooking. In addition, I recommend starting your morning with zing and a dash. Add the juice of half a lemon and a generous sprinkle of cayenne pepper to a cup of hot water.

Drink More Clean Water

Drinking eight or more glasses of pure water will help support hormone balance. Your liver plays a key role in hormone production and metabolism. If your kidneys are water deprived, your liver has to pitch in and help the kidneys do their job, thereby compromising its efficiency. Also, dehydration can create an imbalance of minerals, which can contribute to hormone imbalance. Be leery of pure water packaged in xenoestrogen-leeching plastic bottles. Put a filter on your water tap or choose water bottled in glass.

Beware of Foods That Act as Sexual Vampires

If you are thinking of setting the stage for sex with a romantic dinner of steak, twice-baked potatoes, and a bottle of wine, think again. That meal is more likely to have you and your partner semicomatose on the couch with your pants unbuttoned . . . and not in a let-me-get-ready-for-action kind of way. Look at what happened to Paulo and Pam:

> Pam and I had been going through a sexual dry spell for close to a year when her 39th birthday came around. I thought a special occasion is the perfect chance to get us both back in the groove, so I asked my mother to keep our kids overnight. I took Pam to a romantic little Italian restaurant famous for its homemade lasagna. We drank a great bottle of red wine with dinner, and when I was about to pay the check, our waiter gave us a piece of chocolate raspberry cheesecake on the house. Our dinner was delicious, but instead of setting the stage for action when we got home, I was only able to manage a few kisses and a hug before I was snoring away. Pam said she didn't mind because her stomach felt so full she was afraid she might throw up if she moved around too much. Unfortunately, the kids were back before breakfast, so we blew that chance to get out of our sexual rut.

It is sad enough when sexual expectations get derailed by work or child responsibilities, but when food is the culprit, a missed sexual opportunity is a downright tragedy. Unknowingly, Paulo and Pam had chosen a meal certain to interfere with their plans for a sexy birthday celebration. And if they continue to lift forks overflowing with heavy foods high in saturated fats, they will be digging themselves deeper into their sexual rut. If you want to eat your way to great sex, you need to immediately eliminate consumption of the following:

- **Fast foods:** If you are in the habit of eating drive-through meals, processed meats, nightly nachos, and beer or sugary doughnuts washed down with multiple cups of coffee, your poor eating habits are interfering with hormone balance and are smothering your sex drive. The odds are that you are also overweight, with a good bit of extra fat hanging around your middle, making you even more estrogen dominant. No wonder you don't have the energy or desire for sex.

- **Foods high in saturated, refined polyunsaturated, or trans fats:** Saturated fats are found in fried foods and high-fat meats such as pork sausage, spareribs, bologna, liverwurst, bacon, ham, frankfurters, and bratwurst. Refined polyunsaturated and trans fats are commonly found in commercial salad dressings, french fries, potato chips, butter, margarine, lard, the shortening in most cookies and pastries, and cream. Over time, too much of these unhealthy fats can clog arteries and prevent adequate flow of blood in the genital region. *Note:* Many foward-thinking food manufacturers have eliminated trans fats as an ingredient. For a healthy alternative, look for "0 Trans fats" on the label.

- **Simple carbohydrates:** Overconsumption of the "white" group, such as sugar, white flour, Idaho potatoes, and white rice, has been found to raise blood sugar levels and stimulate insulin release, which then negatively impacts hormone balance.

Remember the Guidelines for Caffeine and Alcohol

Caffeinated and alcoholic beverages usually get a bad rap regarding their influence on hormone balance and overall health, but there are exceptions. Studies show that daily consumption of one cup of java and one glass of red wine for women or two for men can be beneficial to your health. Here's the scoop:

- **Caffeine:** Studies have shown that drinking two cups of coffee a day may increase estrogen levels and overstimulate the adrenal glands. In a clinical trial involving approximately five hundred women between the ages of 36 and 45, women who consumed more than one cup of coffee a day had significantly higher levels of estrogen during the early follicular phase of their menstrual cycle. Those who consumed at least 500 mg of caffeine daily, the equivalent of four to five cups of coffee, had nearly 70 percent more estrogen than women who consumed less than 100 mg of caffeine daily.

  On the flip side, nutritional studies have found that coffee is the number one source of antioxidants in the American diet. As you just learned, antioxidants have many health benefits. Fruits and vegetables are the richest and most preferred source of antioxidants. But if you can't think of starting your morning without the jolt of coffee, keep it to one cup, then switch to decaffeinated coffee or green tea, another great source of antioxidants.

- **Alcohol:** Many people use alcohol to loosen themselves up in anticipation of having sex, and some people believe that alcohol is an aphrodisiac. Recent medical studies have shown that when consumed in moderation, red wine can contribute to heart health. But the actual sexual and health effects of alcohol are complicated, and there are many serious negative sexual consequences of drinking too much and drinking too often. Let's start by understanding how alcohol influences sexual arousal and response:

- In small amounts, alcohol has been reported to have a positive impact on sexual desire and arousal.
- Research shows that after a few drinks sexual response is reduced.
- In large amounts, alcohol makes sex difficult to impossible.
- As drinking increases, both men and women will experience a reduction in sexual arousal, men may have difficulty getting erections, and both men and women may have difficulty experiencing orgasm.

Now consider the positive and negative impacts that drinking alcoholic beverages can have on your health:

- Red wine is a particularly rich source of two antioxidants chemically named resveratrol and flavonoids. These antioxidants have been proven to have heart-healthy benefits. Resveratrol, found in grape skins and seeds, increases HDL cholesterol and prevents blood clotting. Flavonoids exhibit antioxidant properties that may prevent blood clots and plaque formation in arteries.
- Estrogen is broken down in the liver. If your liver is diseased or overtaxed by the consumption of alcoholic beverages, it will be unable to efficiently and effectively break down the estrogen circulating in your body, thereby contributing to or worsening an underlying condition of estrogen dominance.

If you do not already drink alcohol, don't start. You have plenty of other options to loosen you up and add antioxidants to your diet. If you already drink alcohol and want to continue, drink red wine in moderation: one 4-ounce glass of red wine per day for women and one to two 4-ounce glasses for men.

Your Daily Recipe for Better Sex

Did you notice that a number of foods popped up in more than one sexually stimulating category? These are your dietary sex superstars. If you are a bit overwhelmed at how to pull this constellation of stars into focus, this table should help.

Sexy Food Superstar	Health, Sex, and Hormone Benefits
Flaxseeds, sesame seeds, flaxseed oil	• Essential fatty acid: ↑ Testosterone • Lignans: promote estrogen balance • L-arginine: ↑ nitric oxide, blood flow to ↑ penile and clitoral response • Omega-3 fatty acid: ↑ sexual stamina and orgasm potential • ↑ good cholesterol (HDL), promote heart health, improve circulation to the genitals
Nuts and seeds: almonds, peanuts, sesame oil, pecans, pistachio nuts, cashews, hazelnuts, macadamia nuts, Brazil nuts, sesame seeds	• Zinc: ↑ testosterone • Essential fatty acid: ↑ testosterone • L-arginine: ↑ nitric oxide, blood flow to ↑ penile and clitoral response • ↑ good cholesterol (HDL), promote heart health, improve circulation to the genitals
Dark leafy vegetables: broccoli, spinach, Brussels sprouts, kale, turnips, collard and mustard greens	• Essential fatty acid: ↑ testosterone • Cruciferous vegetables w/indole-3-carbinol: ↓ "bad" estrogen • L-arginine: ↑ nitric oxide, blood flow to ↑ penile and clitoral response • Antioxidants: ↑ circulation, sexual performance, and response
Oily fish: salmon, herring, mackerel, sardines	• Essential fatty acid: ↑ testosterone • L-arginine: ↑ nitric oxide, blood flow to ↑ penile and clitoral response

(continued)

Sexy Food Superstar	Health, Sex, and Hormone Benefits
	• ↑ good cholesterol (HDL), promote heart health, improve circulation to the genitals
Liver	• Zinc: ↑ testosterone • Vitamin A: ↑ testosterone
Citrus fruits	• D-limonene: ↓ estrogen • Antioxidants: ↑ circulation, sexual performance, and response
Whole grains	• Zinc: ↑ testosterone • Insoluble fiber: ↓ estrogen

A Simple Checklist for Sexy Eating

If you are going to eat sexy for life, grocery shopping and food preparation have to be easy. The following checklist and table provide simple at-a-glance guides of what to eat to increase your sexual gusto and trim down that gut. No matter your age or underlying hormonal condition, both women and men should:

✓ Eat three meals every day.
  • Have a 4- to 6-ounce portion of protein with every meal.
    - Four to five times per week, eat oily fish, including salmon, herring, mackerel, and sardines.
    - Four to five times per week, eat phytoestrogen-rich sources of protein, including tofu, tempeh, soy milk, and textured soy protein. Soy protein is also found in many "meat analog" products, such as soy sausages, burgers, franks, and cold cuts, as well as soy yogurts and cheese, all of which are intended as substitutes for their animal-based counterparts.
    - Eat liver once per week.
    - Alternate with other fish, mollusks, shellfish, poultry, lean beef, eggs, and dried beans (including lentils).

- Eat three to five servings of vegetables and fruits every day.
- Have one serving of soluble fiber (oatmeal, oat bran, kidney beans, apples, pears, psyllium, barley, prunes) and two servings of insoluble fiber (whole grains, whole-wheat breads, barley, couscous, brown rice, whole-grain breakfast cereals, wheat bran, seeds, carrots, cucumbers, zucchini, celery, tomatoes) every day.
- We haven't talked about this before, but you are going to need strong bones for your increasingly active sex life. Include two servings per day of calcium-rich foods, including yogurt, collards, skim milk, spinach, cheese, cottage cheese, canned salmon, and black-eyed peas.

✓ Cook and season with virgin or extra-virgin olive oil.

✓ Liberally use flaxseeds and flaxseed oil as a seasoning for vegetables and salads, as well as an add-in to yogurt, cottage cheese, and smoothies.

✓ Eat healthy snacks between meals when hungry.

- Have 2 or 3 ounces of raw or lightly roasted nuts or seeds every day as a snack.
- Eat a piece of fresh fruit every day.
- Enjoy one or two dark chocolate Hershey kisses two or three times per week.

✓ Drink water, water, water.

- Try hot water with the juice of half a lemon and a sprinkle of cayenne pepper.
- If you just have to have coffee, limit yourself to one cup per day; green tea or decaffeinated coffee is preferable.

Now let's fine-tune this food plan to coincide with your individual hormone balance concerns:

Hormone Condition	Choose to Eat
• ♀ who are estrogen dominant or estrogen deficient; e.g., any ♀ over 35 • ♀ who have had a partial or complete hysterectomy • ♀ or ♂ who have been 10 pounds or more overweight for more than one year • ♀ or ♂ chronically exposed to environmental xenoestrogens	Phytoestrogen-rich foods: soy products, including soybeans, soy milk, tofu, tempeh, textured vegetable protein, roasted soybeans, miso, edamame Cruciferous vegetables: broccoli, asparagus, cauliflower, spinach, Brussels sprouts, celery, alfalfa, beet root, kale, cabbage, parsley root, radishes, turnips, collards, mustard greens Citrus fruits: oranges, grapefruits, tangerines, lemons, limes, tangelos Insoluble fiber: whole grains, whole-wheat breads, barley, couscous, brown rice, whole-grain cereals, wheat bran, seeds, carrots, cucumbers, zucchini, celery, tomatoes Lignans: ground or milled flaxseeds, sesame seeds, flaxseed oil
• ♂ or ♀ who are testosterone deficient • ♂ over 40 • ♀ who are perimenopausal or menopausal • ♀ who have had a partial or complete hysterectomy	Foods rich in zinc: oysters and other mollusks, beef, liver, poultry, shrimp and crab, nuts and seeds, whole grains, tofu, peanuts and peanut butter, lentils, yogurt, milk Foods rich in essential fatty acid: flaxseed oil, flaxseeds, flaxseed meal, hempseed oil, hempseeds, walnuts, pumpkin seeds, olive oil (extra-virgin or virgin), olives, avocados, almonds, peanuts, sesame oil, pecans, pistachio nuts, cashews, hazelnuts, macadamia nuts, Brazil nuts, sesame seeds, some dark leafy green vegetables

Hormone Condition	Choose to Eat
	(kale, spinach, purslane, mustard greens, collards, etc.), canola oil (cold-pressed and unrefined), soybean oil, wheat germ oil, oily fish (salmon, mackerel, sardines, anchovies, albacore tuna)
	Foods rich in vitamin A: liver, egg yolks, full-fat milk, cod liver oil
• ♂ or ♀ suffering from heart disease, circulatory problems, and/or decreased sexual pleasure, performance, or sensation	Foods rich in L-arginine: nuts and seeds (peanuts, almonds, walnuts, hazelnuts, Brazil nuts, cashews, pecans, pistachio nuts, flaxseeds, sunflower seeds), granola, oatmeal, canned tuna, salmon, cod, halibut, shrimp, poultry, dried beans, chickpeas, garlic, eggs, green vegetables, dark chocolate
	Foods rich in antioxidants: citrus fruits (oranges, grapefruits, tangelos, tangerines), cruciferous vegetables (broccoli, cauliflower, green leafy vegetables, Brussels sprouts), tomatoes, beets, bell peppers, berries, red grapes. *Note:* dark chocolate, coffee, and red wine in moderation.
	Healthy fats and good cholesterol: foods high in soluble fiber (oatmeal, oat bran, kidney beans, apples, pears, psyllium, barley, prunes), walnuts and almonds, fish high in omega-3 fatty acids, olive oil
	Cayenne, ginger, and garlic

In Appendix A, grocery lists are matched with meal plans and recipes. Follow my food plan for just two weeks and your hormone balance, improved body, and recharged sexual appetite will begin to take on roots at a cellular level.

Want to turn this dietary foundation into a springboard of healthy, sexy hormones? In Chapter 8 you'll learn which natural supplements can gently, yet quite effectively, boost and balance hormone levels. If you have been waiting for the secret to restoring youthful sexual fireworks, just keep turning the page.

8

Step 2: Herbal Medicine Puts You
in the Mood to Go Horizontal

When 45-year-old Erica sat down in my office, she was at the end of her rope:

> I have gone up two pants sizes in just two years and I swear I am eating less, not more. I tried keeping a food diary, but I forgot where I put it, just like I am always forgetting where I leave my purse, keys, and glasses. I am constantly snapping at my husband, Constantine, and he is lucky if we have sex once a month. Even then, I am sure he can tell I am just not into it. It's sad, because when we were in our 20s and 30s, sex was a huge part of our lives. I had a bureau full of incredible lingerie, and Constantine kept a ready supply of mood music, candles, and warming ointments. I am desperate. Is there any hope you can help me get my body, my mind, and my sex drive back?

Many women, like Erica, have restored youthful sexual vitality by pairing a hormone-balancing diet with herbal supplements. In contrast to synthetic HRT or even BHRT, herbal medicine takes a more gradual and gentle approach to boosting and balancing sex hormones. While herbs can take a little longer than BHRT to take effect, once they have sufficiently built up in your system, the results are wonderful. More exciting, their positive impact on your sexuality and overall wellness can work for a lifetime.

Herbal medicine, technically called phytotherapy, is the science of using plants, either in whole-food form or in the form of standardized extracts and supplements, for healing purposes. This approach is definitely not "new age" medicine. In fact, the age-old science of herbal medicine is the root of modern pharmacology.

For centuries, herbal remedies have been used in China and India, as well as in Native American cultures. In the last two decades, herbal medicine's popularity within the United States has skyrocketed. In 1993, David Eisenberg and other researches from Beth Israel Hospital and Harvard Medical School published a landmark study in the *New England Journal of Medicine* documenting the increasing usage of herbal remedies in the United States.[1] In 1997, surveys indicated that over 40 percent of Americans were self-treating with an herbal remedy, and it has been estimated that over 80 percent of the world's population embrace phytotherapuetic, or botanical, medicine as part of a comprehensive approach to primary care.[2]

I have long been a proponent of herbal medicine, and Randy was a compounding pharmacist with in-depth training in pharmacognosy (the study of plants as medicine) before attending medical school. We merged our individual expertise to develop the following unique and natural approach to boosting and balancing your hormones.

Plant-Based Hormones Can Help Restore Hormone Balance

For anyone who wants to restore hormone balance naturally but who can't find or can't afford BHRT, plant-based hormones, or phytohormones, are an excellent alternative. In the last chapter, you learned how foods containing phytoestrogens can mimic the estrogen once produced by the ovaries. Now I am suggesting taking this approach to another level. Plant-derived hormone supplements can build on that nutritional foundation to stabilize optimum hormone levels and snowball your sex drive.

Some plants contain bioactive molecules that resemble the molecular structure of the sex hormones produced by the human ovaries or testes. When introduced into your body, phytohormones weakly bind to hormone receptors, promoting the same physiologic response as estrogen, progesterone, or testosterone. Unlike the dangerous side effects produced by the different molecular structure of synthetic hormones, plant-derived supplements are safe because of their unique modulating effect. The plant molecule adaptively works with your body to respond to current hormone levels, so you never get too much or too little. For instance, if your body is estrogen dominant, a phytoestrogen molecule will block the negative effects of excess estrogen; alternately, when estrogen levels decline during the perimenopausal or menopausal years, phytoestrogens can double for missing estrogen molecules to moderate the negative effects of estrogen deficiency.

Like BHRT, I do not advocate a one-size-fits-all approach to herbal hormone balancing. Most product package directions allow for a range of dosing, such as 200 to 400 mg or two to four capsules per day. I recommend starting with a low dose, and if symptoms of hormone imbalance persist after two weeks, gradually increase your dosage toward the upper end of the range.

Certain vitamins and other nutritional supplements work synergistically with phytohormones to stabilize optimum hormone balance. This chapter provides specific recommendations that correspond with different types of hormone imbalance— for example, estrogen dominance or deficiency.

Finally, phytohormones are at most only 2 to 4 percent as potent as the hormones produced by your body or bioidentical hormones. In most cases, it takes time for these herbal remedies to build up and have an effect in the body. Noticeable differences in your libido and feelings of sexual arousal and pleasure will typically occur in four to six weeks, but in some cases you may need to be patient for four months.

Oops . . . I almost lost you with that time frame, didn't I? I encourage you to not get impatient. You did not jump from being 25 years old to 40 or 50 overnight, so doesn't it make sense that a gradual and gentle approach for rejuvenating your sexuality may take a little time to be effective? This approach is not readying you for a sexual sprint; it is preparing your body for a lifetime sexual marathon.

If You Are Estrogen Dominant

As discussed in Chapter 5, if estrogen dominance has your sex drive in a straitjacket, you can safely use over-the-counter (OTC) bioidentical progesterone cream to help neutralize your underlying condition. Though not as potent as the bioidentical version, chaste berry (Vitex agnus castus) and licorice (Glycyrrhiza glabra) are phytoprogesterone supplements that can also stand in for the progesterone molecules your body is lacking. Certain vitamins and other nutritional supplements work to help accelerate your body's offloading of its unhealthy extra estrogen.

Chaste Berry

Chaste berry is widely used in Europe and is approved by the German Commission E, a governmental regulatory agency founded in 1978 to evaluate the usefulness of herbs as medicine, to treat hormonal imbalances and abnormal bleeding as well as bloating, mood swings, food cravings, and premenstrual bleeding. In medieval Europe, chaste berry was popular among celibate clergymen for its purported ability to reduce unwanted sexual libido, yielding the common name "monk's pepper." In ancient Greece, young women celebrating the festival of Demeter wore chaste berry blossoms to show that they were remaining chaste in honor of the goddess.

Contrary to its name and reputation, chaste berry actually has a libido-*boosting* effect, but you must have your ovaries for it to work! This supplement acts on the hypothalamus and pituitary glands to increase luteinizing hormone (LH) and mildly inhibit follicle-stimulating hormone (FSH). The result is a progesterone-like shift in the ratio of estrogen and progesterone.

Note: This is not a fast-acting herb. Results may take three to four months.

Licorice Root

Clinical studies have found that licorice root supplements decrease symptoms of PMS and menopause, including mild depression. Licorice root inhibits an enzyme that breaks down progesterone, thereby raising progesterone and lowering estrogen levels. Recent laboratory studies found that licorice root may also improve memory and cognition.[3]

Despite these promising findings, there is an ongoing debate in the scientific community regarding the value and side effects of licorice root products. People who regularly consume large amounts of licorice (more than 20 g/day) may inadvertently raise blood levels of the hormone aldosterone, which can cause serious side effects, including headache, high blood pressure, and heart problems.

Caution: Avoid supplements containing licorice root if you have high blood pressure, heart rhythm irregularities, or kidney disease.

Calcium D-Glucarate

Calcium D-glucarate is a natural substance that promotes the body's detoxification of extra estrogen and supports hormonal balance. Calcium D-glucarate inhibits the reabsorption of estrogen-like toxins into the bloodstream, allowing them to be excreted in the feces. I recommend taking 1,000 to 2,000 mg twice daily.

Diindolymethane

Diindolymethane (DIM) is a phytonutrient akin to the indole-3-carbinol (I3C) found in cruciferous vegetables. DIM has unique hormonal benefits. It supports the activity of enzymes that improve estrogen metabolism by increasing the levels of 2-hydroxyestrone, the "good" estrogen. I have found that DIM helps with PMS symptoms, fat loss, and healthy estrogen metabolism. I recommend that women take 200 to 300 mg once daily.

If You Are Estrogen Deficient

Stefanie, a dynamic 51-year-old freelance writer and mother of four, spoke accusingly:

> Either the manufacturers of the bioidentical progesterone and estriol creams I buy in the health food store have changed their formula or those other supplements I have been taking are not as strong as they used to be. My hot flashes, night sweats, and mood swings are back with a vengeance, and my sex drive has dissipated to a new low. I am miserable and I can assure you that my husband is more than pissed.

"I understand your frustration, but your problem is not a change in the strength of what you have been taking," I responded. "You started that regimen five years ago. Your hormone profile today is undoubtedly very different than it was then. When did you last have a period?"

"Well, that is one thing I am grateful for," Stefanie told me. "I haven't had a period for sixteen months and I most definitely don't miss the hassle."

"Stefanie," I counseled, "not having a period for over a year means that you are now officially menopausal. What your body previously needed to restore its hormone balance is no longer enough. Your recurring symptoms are a signal that your body needs something more; it needs an additional estrogen boost."

"No way," Stefanie countered. "I read how those estrogen drugs increase a woman's risk of heart disease and cancer. I saw Oprah's shows on the benefits of prescription bioidentical hormones, but she can afford to pay out-of-pocket for a doctor's consultation and a customized treatment regimen. I can't. So am I just screwed?"

"Absolutely not," I said. "There are some excellent plant-based alternatives that capture the benefits of estrogen without the risk of side effects. Just as wonderful, a month's supply will cost you little more than a large pizza."

Lab work and a personal hormone-level profile is the definitive method to determine if and to what degree your body is estrogen deficient. Without this testing, however, the following parameters will indicate whether you need more estrogen:

A. If OTC bioidentical progesterone and estriol creams worked for a while but now your symptoms are back

B. If you are perimenopausal or menopausal and are experiencing vaginal dryness, vaginal atrophy, and/or painful intercourse and OTC bioidentical progesterone and estriol creams are not working

C. If you have had a partial or complete hysterectomy and OTC bioidentical progesterone and estriol creams are not working

To mimic nature and get the most benefit from a supplemental approach to hormone restoration, perimenopausal women should take phytoestrogen supplements cyclically: three weeks on and one week off. Menopausal women can take them every day. Women must always balance natural estrogenic supplementation with OTC bioidentical progesterone cream. This is a must. Chaste berry and licorice root are not strong enough to balance estrogen supplementation on their own.

There are several potent and well-researched phytoestrogens available in capsules, creams, and tinctures. Follow the package directions for safe dosage. Some women find that they respond to a certain phytoestrogen alone or in combination better than others. Your options are explained next.

8-Prenylnaringenin and 7-Hydroxymatairesinol

An extract of the female flower of the hops plant contains a potent phytonutrient known as 8-prenylnaringenin (8-PN). Controlled clinical studies have shown that most menopausal women who take 8-PN experience a rapid and significant reduction in hot flashes and other physical discomforts related to estrogen deficiency. In fact, German investigators testing 8-PN in animal studies found that its estrogenic activity was higher than that of any other phytoestrogenic plant.

Research suggests that a phytoestrogen derived from Norway spruce with the chemical name 7-hydroxymatairesinol (7-HMR) reduces hot flashes, night sweats, and insomnia by about 50 percent.

Genistein and Daidzein

Genistein and daidzein are two of the most extensively studied phytoestrogens. In one medical study published in 2003, Cotter and colleagues reported that "dietary supplementation with 54 mg/day of genistein is as effective as HRT without causing the associated side effects." Other medical scientists report that treatment with 54 mg/day of genistein safely decreases hot flashes by up to 30 percent. Finally, genistein in combination with daidzein has been shown to have beneficial effects for bones, brain function, and the cardiovascular system.[4]

Black Cohosh

Black cohosh, a member of the buttercup family, is a perennial plant that is native to North America. Native Americans have used black cohosh as a treatment for rheumatism (arthritis and muscle pain) and also for menopausal symptoms including hot flashes, night sweats, and vaginal dryness.

Clinical study results are mixed on black cohosh's effectiveness. Studies in Europe have found this phytoestrogen to be so effective that a black cohosh extract called Remifemin is commonly prescribed as an alternative to synthetic hormone replacement. In 2004, the North American Menopause Society (NAMS) added its stamp of approval to the use of black cohosh. In fact, it recommended black cohosh as a first-line approach. Its position statement reads, in part: "In women who need relief for mild [hot flashes and night sweats], NAMS recommends first considering lifestyle changes, either alone or combined with a nonprescription remedy, such as the dietary isoflavone black cohosh."[5] In contrast, a National Center for Complimentary Medicine (NCCA)–funded study found that black cohosh, whether used alone or with other botanicals, failed to relieve hot flashes and night sweats in women during or after menopause.[6]

Dong Quai

Dong quai, also known as Chinese angelica, has been used for thousands of years in traditional Chinese, Korean, and Japanese medicine. It remains one of the most popular plants in Chinese medicine, and it is used primarily to treat female gynecologic problems. Dong quai is often called the "female ginseng" based on its use for painful menstruation or pelvic pain, recovery from childbirth or illness, and fatigue/low vitality. It is also given for strengthening *xue* (loosely translated as "the blood"), cardiovascular conditions/high blood pressure, inflammation, headache, infections, and nerve pain.

In the late 1800s, an extract of dong quai called *Eumenol* became popular in Europe as a treatment for gynecological complaints. Recently, interest in dong quai has resurged due to its popularity among menopausal women.

Caution: Dong quai should not be used by people with bleeding disorders, excessive menstrual bleeding, diarrhea, abdominal bloating, or during infections such as colds or flu. People taking blood thinners (anticoagulants) such as warfarin should not use dong quai. Dong quai can cause photosensitivity, so people should limit sun exposure and wear sunblock.

Red Clover (Trifolium pratense)

Red clover, a wild plant used as grazing food for cattle and other livestock, has also been used to treat a wide array of conditions. These have included cancer, mastitis (inflammation of the breast), joint disorders, jaundice, bronchitis, spasmodic coughing, asthma, and skin inflammations, such as psoriasis and eczema. Red clover is thought to "purify" the blood by promoting urine and mucus production, improving circulation, and stimulating the secretion of bile.

Recently, red clover's rich phytoestrogenic properties have gained attention. Studies have shown promise in using red clover to treat menopausal symptoms such as hot flashes, cardiovascular health, and the bone loss associated with osteoporosis.

In addition to boosting estrogen levels with phytoestrogens, women who are estrogen deficient should also take vitamin E.

Vitamin E

Vitamin E has been found to relieve hot flashes and night sweats, as well as breast tenderness and vaginal dryness. It improves the blood supply to the vagina. Vitamin E oil can be used topically to treat thinning and inflammation of the vaginal wall that can occur with the onset of menopause.

Nutritional Supplements Every Woman Needs

Many nutritional experts agree that even if you ate a healthy diet including raw and organic fruits and vegetables every day, you could not consume enough of the foods to supply your body with all the needed vitamins and minerals. According to the *Dietary Guidelines for Americans 2005*, adults are often deficient in:

- Calcium
- Magnesium
- Vitamin A (as carotenoids)
- Vitamin C
- Vitamin E

Multivitamins

I recommend that everyone take a top-quality multivitamin every day to begin to fill in nutritional gaps, including a dietary insufficiency of vitamin A. Choose a multivitamin that includes fish oil.

Note: Although a multivitamin will contain vitamins B, C, and E, your body needs more of these vitamins than the multi will provide. Consequently, I recommend additional supplementation.

Calcium–Magnesium Combo

Most women and men find it difficult to get 1,200 to 1,500 mg of calcium from their diet. As a rule, I recommend a calcium–magnesium combination supplement.

Magnesium helps the body eliminate excess estrogen. For women, magnesium levels tend to fall at certain times during the menstrual cycle. These shifts can upset an optimum calcium–magnesium ratio. In proper balance, the body better absorbs and assimilates the calcium it needs and allows calcium to migrate out of tissues and organs where it doesn't belong.

Without magnesium, calcium may be not fully utilized. Underabsorption of calcium can lead to menstrual cramps. Similar to a vitamin E deficiency, when the body does not have enough magnesium to support calcium absorption, many women report PMS symptoms, such as mood swings, fatigue, headaches, and sleeplessness. I recommend that you take a calcium–magnesium supplement that combines these minerals in a ratio of two parts calcium (1,500 mg) to one part magnesium (750 mg).

B-Complex Vitamins

The B vitamins, such as B1, B2, B3, B5, B6, B12, and folate, do a lot within your body to support overall health and hormone balance. Although many people consume foods fortified with vitamin B, the typical American diet that is high in processed, cooked, and microwavable food provides only a fraction of the B vitamins we need for good health. Because these vitamins are vital to a vigorous and long life, not getting them can lead to serious problems. B vitamins are easily flushed out of the body, and people on weight-loss diets, alcoholics, or those who take antibiotics or seizure drugs are even more inclined to have vitamin B deficiency.

Because the B vitamins work together to perform such vital tasks at the cellular level, I recommend you take the entire B-complex, not just one or two of the vitamins. To treat symptoms of hormone imbalance, take 100 mg of B-complex twice a day.

Vitamin C

This is the healing vitamin. It helps to mend wounds and burns and maintains collagen (it is sometimes called the antiwrinkle vitamin). Since the need for collagen regeneration increases with age, so does the need for vitamin C. It also helps the adrenal glands and the immune system, which needs more help as we enter midlife and menopause. I recommend 1,000 units of vitamin C daily.

Vitamin D3

A deficiency in vitamin D3 has been linked to an increased risk of osteoporosis, depression, diabetes, heart disease, and cancer of the breast, prostate, and colon. Other symptoms include fatigue, hair loss, and weight gain. I recommend 1,000 IU of vitamin D3 daily.

How Safe Are Natural Supplements?

Until recently, government oversight and consumer protection for dietary supplements was very limited. But new regulations contained within the Federal Food, Drug, and Cosmetic Act give the FDA the authority to oversee the manufacture of domestic- and foreign-made dietary supplements, including herbal supplements.

Dietary supplements don't need to go through the rigorous review process that new drugs must undergo before being approved by the FDA. But these new regulations aim to improve safety by requiring supplement manufacturers to follow certain manufacturing practices and to ensure that supplements contain what their labels claim and are free of contaminants. The FDA is responsible for monitoring the safety of supplements after they're on the market and enforcing action against unsafe products. These new regulations will be phased in over a three-year period. By June 2010, all supplement manufacturers should meet these requirements.

In addition, the herb and supplement industry has its own organizations that regulate product manufacturing. The American Herbal Products Association has created a code of ethics and a safety handbook. The Natural Nutritional Foods Association's (NNFA) mission is to ensure truth in labeling and packaging. When purchasing any herbal product, you should inspect the label to make sure it includes the following:

- The name of the herbal supplement, such as L-arginine.
- The net quantity of contents, such as 100 tablets.
- A Supplements Facts panel that includes a listing and amounts of active ingredients.
- A listing of other ingredients, such as amino acids, for which no daily values have been established.
- The name and address of the manufacturer, packer, or distributor.
- The U.S. Pharmacopeia's "USP Dietary Supplement Verified" seal, which indicates the supplement has met certain manufacturing standards. These standards include testing the product for uniformity, cleanliness, and freedom from

environmental contaminants, such as lead, mercury, or
drugs. Other groups that certify herbal supplements include
ConsumerLab.com, Good Housekeeping, and NSF
International. Although each group takes a slightly different
approach, the goal is to certify that herbal supplements meet
a certain standard.

Be extremely cautious about herbal supplements manufactured outside the United States. Many European herbs are highly regulated and standardized. But toxic ingredients and prescription drugs have been found in some herbal supplements manufactured in other countries.

Get Back That Sizzle

The table below recaps the information in this chapter to help you determine the phytohormones and natural supplements you can begin taking to restore your feelings of desire and get back your much-missed sizzle:

If You Are	You Need	Effects	Notes/ Contraindications
Estrogen Dominant • ♀ over 35 having regular periods • ♀ who have been 10 pounds or more over-	To Balance 1. OTC bioidentical progesterone cream is a must; may add: 2. Chaste berry or	A positive shift in the body's estrogen to progesterone ratio to ↑ libido and eliminate other symptoms of estrogen dominance	A recap of symptoms of estrogen dominance: ✓ Decreased libido ✓ Weight gain ✓ Hot flashes ✓ Night sweats ✓ Worsened PMS

If You Are	You Need	Effects	Notes/ Contraindications
weight for over a year and who are suffering from two or more symptoms of estrogen dominance • ♂ who have been 10 pounds or more overweight for over a year and who are suffering from two or more symptoms of estrogen dominance	3. Licorice root To ↑ Off-Loading of E 1. Calcium D-glucarate 2. DIM		✓ Sleep disturbances ✓ Mood swings/ depression ✓ Foggy thinking ✓ Fatigue, burned-out feeling ✓ Headaches/ migraines ✓ Bloating ✓ Osteoporosis ✓ Fibrocystic breasts Do not take any supplement containing licorice root if you have high blood pressure, heart rhythm irregularities, or kidney disease.
Estrogen Deficient • ♀ who are perimenopausal or menopausal and experiencing vaginal dryness, thinning of the vaginal walls,	To Boost OTC estriol cream + one of the following: 1. 8-PN 2. HMR 3. Genistein and daidzein 4. Black cohosh 5. Dong quai 6. Red clover	Improved vaginal lubrication and healthy thickening of the vaginal walls	Any form of estrogen supplementation should always be balanced with progesterone, preferably OTC bioidentical progesterone cream. Chaste berry and licorice root also help to neutralize

(continued)

If You Are	You Need	Effects	Notes/ Contraindications
and/or painful intercourse • ♀ who have had a partial or complete hysterectomy			estrogen's propensity to promote cell growth, but they are not as potent.
For Every Woman	To Support Overall Health 1. Multivitamin with fish oil 2. Calcium–magnesium supplement 3. B-complex 4. Vitamin C 5. Vitamin D3		

9

Natural Testosterone Enhancers
Lift the Limp and Lustless

At 52, Robert was a highly visible city councilman, church deacon, and father of three boys in college. He was a man who prided himself on being in charge, so when he called me to talk about his sex life, he did so with obvious discomfort:

> It embarrasses me to be speaking to a woman about my sexual problems, but I am at my wits' end and need help. Since my wife, Erica, had been on your diet and taking the supplements you recommended, she has turned into a wild cat in the bedroom. I used to have to beg her for Saturday night sex; now, she wants to make love once or twice a day. The truth is I can't keep up. My doctor wrote me a prescription for Viagra, but it gave me horrible headaches and diarrhea. Do you have anything natural that you recommend for men with these problems?

Like Robert, many men are embarrassed by sexual dysfunction, but the issue is not their manhood; it is an age-related medical condition. The good news is that erectile dysfunction (ED) and low libido are quite reversible without side effect–ridden drugs like Viagra. Phytotherapy, or plant-based medicine, has been medically proven to restore male sex drive and strong, firm erections.

Men Need an Offense and a Defense

Age-related decline in testosterone production is a problem for both sexes, but it is most prevalent in men. One issue is that the testes can't pump out as much testosterone. Another is that as the years go by, levels of an enzyme called aromatase begin to rise. Aromatase converts testosterone to estrogen, so more aromatase means additional pillaging of a man's much-needed testosterone supply.

Certain herbs offensively boost levels of free testosterone while defensively blocking the conversion, or aromatization, of testosterone to estrogen. Herbal medicine can get you ready to score!

Note: The following herbs will also help women suffering from testosterone deficiency, but because the female body needs only one-tenth the amount of testosterone as the male body, the required dosage will be sufficiently less.

Maca Tuber (Peruvian Ginseng)
When Spanish explorers arrived in Peru during the sixteenth century, they noticed that their livestock—particularly their horses—were becoming weak and unable to reproduce. This was probably due to the altitudes of the Peruvian highlands, an area where mountains reach fifteen thousand feet. High altitudes can

cause female animals to produce inadequate amounts of estrogen, hampering fertility.

The Incan diet of the time consisted largely of maca. The Incas used both tubers and tops, but especially tubers. They advised the Spaniards to feed maca tubers to the ailing and infertile horses. So impressed were the Spaniards with the recovery of their animals, and the strength and virility of the Incan people, that reports back to the royal court included raves over this humble tuber. Maca soon became a valuable commodity.

Maca tuber's reputation as a natural way to boost virility and fertility is growing fast in North America. Clinical trials performed on men have shown that maca extracts can heighten libido and improve semen quality.[1] For women, maca tuber has been shown to regulate the entire endocrine system and help balance hormone levels to eliminate hot flashes and depression while also increasing libido and sexual stamina.[2]

In 2008, medical scientists at Massachusetts General Hospital investigated maca tuber as a treatment for sexual dysfunction in women and men taking a selective serotonin reuptake inhibitor (SSRI) class of antidepressant drugs, such as Prozac, Zoloft, and Paxil. Subjects experienced a significant improvement in libido.[3]

Finally, maca tuber is a food as well as a plant-based medicine. The maca plant is brimming with major and trace minerals, vitamins, alkaloids, and essential fatty acids. It contains more than sixty phytonutrients and thirty-one trace minerals and is high in protein, fiber, calcium, magnesium, and vitamins A, B1, B2, B3, B12, C, D, and E.

Muira Puama

Research indicates that muira puama (also known as potency wood) is one of the best herbs to use for ED or lack of libido. This shrub is native to Brazil and has long been used as a powerful aphrodisiac and nerve stimulant in South American folk medicine. A recent study has validated its safety and effectiveness in improving libido and sexual function in some patients.[4]

At the Institute of Sexology in Paris, France, Jacques Waynberg investigated muira puama's effectiveness in a clinical study with 262 patients complaining of lack of sexual desire and the inability to attain or maintain an erection. Within two weeks, 62 percent of patients with loss of libido claimed that the treatment had a dynamic effect while 51 percent of patients with erection failures felt that muira puama was of benefit.[5]

Also of interest are recent studies showing that muira puama improved memory and cognitive function in aging mice. Laboratory experiments indicate that muira puama inhibits the breakdown of the neurotransmitter acetylcholine.[6] A declining level of acetylcholine is a hallmark of Alzheimer's disease.

Nettle Root (or Stinging Nettle Root)

Nettle, a leafy plant, grows in most temperate regions. The Latin root of *Urtica*, the genus name, is *uro*, which means "I burn." Small stings caused by the little hairs on the leaves of this plant burn when contact is made with the skin. Its root and leaves are used in herbal medicine.

Nettle root has been shown to increase levels of free testosterone, thereby promoting male vitality and restoring youthful sexual function. The lignan component of nettle root interferes with sexual hormone-binding globulin (SHBG), making it unable to bind to testosterone and pull it out of circulation.[7]

In addition to energizing the libido, stinging nettle root has shown a great deal of promise in treating hypertrophy of the prostate (enlarged prostate), a condition affecting a large proportion of men over the age of 40 that is often a precursor to prostate cancer. The current research shows that constituents of nettle root work by inhibiting the growth of abnormal cells.[8] Interestingly, the same chemicals may have an effect on hair loss, and at least one company has filed a patent for a formula containing stinging nettle root to treat male pattern baldness.

Herbs Restore the Sizzle for Women and Men

Candace and Fran were college roommates when they met and married twin brothers. For twenty-three years, they shared most holidays and summer vacations.

"Do you ever feel like you are just going through the motions?" Candace asked as she lounged in her beach chair digging her toes into the sand. "These days, when Donald and I have sex, I am just plain bored. And no matter what he tries, my having an orgasm during those fifteen to twenty minutes is about as likely as my reading *War and Peace* in a single sitting. Is it the same for you and David?"

"Actually, I have never enjoyed sex more," Fran confided. "Honestly, I am having more fun than I did in the days when David would climb through our dorm room window and he and I would keep you locked out in the hall while we went at it for over an hour. But don't get me wrong. I know exactly how you feel. I was like that for almost three years before I started taking these new supplements."

"What sex toys?" Candace asked in amazement. "Have you been ordering vibrators or kinky videos off the Internet?"

"I said *supplements,* not sex toys," Fran said, laughing. "Seriously, I am not doing anything weird or kinky. After I read an article that linked increased blood flow to the vaginal area with stronger feelings of arousal and pleasure, I went to the health food store and bought these supplements that help my vagina get some much-needed juice."

Candace turned and stared at her old friend as if she had just grown green hair. "Fran, what in the world are you talking about?"

Certain herbs effectively lift libido and improve sexual pleasure and performance by increasing blood flow to the genital area. This section details the ones we most frequently recommend. Note that while some people report feeling sexier in as little as two weeks, you should allow at least four weeks for these pleasure boosters to take full effect.

L-Arginine

L-arginine is one of the more popular supplements for sexual dysfunction for both men and women and is often referred to as nature's Viagra. As you learned in Chapter 7, L-arginine is what the body uses to make the nitric oxide needed to stimulate blood flow to the sexual organs. Clinical studies have shown that men suffering from ED report modest to significant improvements in sexual functioning, including strength of erections and sexual stamina, when taking L-arginine.

In one clinical study 77 women with decreased libido were

given either L-arginine or a placebo. Of the women taking L-arginine, 71 percent showed improvement in sexual desire. They also reported other sexual improvements, including increased frequency of orgasms and improved clitoral sensation.[9] In research published in the *Journal of Sex and Marriage Therapy* in 2001, 108 women of varying ages took either a proprietary L-arginine supplement or a placebo every day for four weeks.[10] At the end of the study, more than two-thirds of pre- and perimenopausal women taking L-arginine reported increased satisfaction with their sex lives. In another study, more than 50 percent of postmenopausal women taking L-arginine said they felt more desire, compared with only 8 percent taking a placebo.[11]

Caution: You should not take L-arginine if you have low blood pressure, heart disease, liver disease, diabetes, genital herpes, or cold sores.

Ginkgo

Ginkgo is best known for its positive effects on memory and cognition. In addition, this herb has been found to improve sexual function in women and men. A clinical study found ginkgo to be effective in treating 84 percent of patients suffering from antidepressant-related sexual dysfunction. In addition to helping patients get back in the mood, participants reported improvement in arousal and strength of orgasm.[12]

Caution: There is some data to suggest that ginkgo can increase bleeding risk, so people who take anticoagulant drugs, have bleeding disorders, or have scheduled surgery or dental procedures should use caution and talk to a health care provider if taking ginkgo.

Ginseng

Ginseng is an umbrella name for several plant species: Asian, American, and Siberian ginseng. Asian ginseng has been shown to improve sexual dysfunction in both men and women and has been used for this purpose in China for thousands of years. Double-blind, placebo-controlled trials have shown that patients taking ginseng experience significantly better sexual function. The active ingredient in Asian ginseng, ginsenoside, facilitates the release of nitric oxide in blood vessels, increasing blood flow to the clitoris and resulting in stronger orgasms.

Caution: Ginseng is usually well tolerated. The most common side effects are headaches and sleep and gastrointestinal problems. Asian ginseng may lower levels of blood sugar; this effect may be seen more in people with diabetes. Therefore, diabetics should consult their physician and use extra caution with Asian ginseng.

Horny Goat Weed

It has a funny name, but horny goat weed is a time-tested aphrodisiac that increases libido in both sexes. Used by Chinese herbalists for more than two thousand years, horny goat weed is a leafy plant that grows in the wild, most abundantly at higher altitudes. While it is not known exactly how horny goat weed works, the plant has long been employed to restore sexual fire, allay fatigue, improve erectile function and fullness, and alleviate symptoms of menopausal discomfort.

Caution: Do not take horny goat weed if you have liver or kidney disease.

Yohimbe

The bark of the herb yohimbe (*Pausinystalia yohimbe*) has historically been used as a folk remedy for low libido, sexual dysfunction, depression, and weight loss. Yohimbe has been used as an aphrodisiac in West Africa for centuries. The extensive folklore surrounding its sexual powers greatly interested European traders who came on expeditions to West Africa. Demand for the bark of yohimbe has been increasing ever since.

Yohimbe is listed in the *Physicians Desk Reference* as a sensual stimulant. It increases blood flow to the genital region for both men and women. It increases reflex excitability in the lower spinal cord, thereby adding to the intensity of the sexual experience. Yohimbe has also been found to make erections harder and help them last longer. The active constituent in the bark is called yohimbine.

Herbal Medicine Versus Viagra

If you are suffering from ED, our herbal approach to get you up and going strong has many advantages over pharmaceutical treatments like Viagra. See the table below for a comparison between Viagra and herbal remedies.

Treatment for Erectile Dysfunction (ED)	Viagra	Herbal Treatments
Mechanism of action	Designed to enhance the body's use of nitric oxide to improve firmness and increase ability to maintain erection.	L-arginine and ginseng: enhances the body's use of nitric oxide. Other herbal treatment choices for ED include: maca, muira puama, nettle root, horny goat weed.

(continued)

Treatment for Erectile Dysfunction (ED)	Viagra	Herbal Treatments
Effectiveness	Very effective but results are short term. Men will be better able to get a firm erection 30–45 minutes after taking pill.	Effects are more cumulative vs. short term. Men will experience firmer and longer-lasting erections after taking herb daily as directed for several weeks. Once baseline level is reached, erections can be achieved with real-time stimulation or event of arousal. No need for preplanning, allows for spontaneity.
Other health benefits	No other health benefits.	Depending on herb: improved libido, increased energy, significant improvement in mood and brain function, alleviation of menopausal symptoms in women.
Side effects	Headache, flushing, stomach upset, nasal stuffiness, diarrhea and dizziness, painful or other urination problems, vision problems, skin rash.	Depending on the herb, no side effects or very few minor side effects. Counter-indications for each herbal remedy described in text.
Typical monthly cost	$120	$30–$50

Help Your "Get Up" Get Going Again

The following tables summarize the herbal formulations we most frequently recommend for men and women seeking to re-ignite their sex drive and add spark to their sexual performance and pleasure. First, we provide our preferred herbal remedies for men wanting to naturally enhance testosterone levels in order to reenergize libido, rejuvenate blood flow to the penis, and improve ability and consistency of erectile function. "Sex-tra" benefits include more energy, improved mood, and a decrease in abdominal body fat and waist circumference.

Second, we list herbs proven to intensify both desire and sexual enjoyment for men and women.

For Men Needing a Testosterone Boost

Herbal Supplement	Source	Effects	Notes
Maca tuber (Peruvian ginseng)	Turnip-like tuber indigenous to the Andean mountains of Peru	↑ libido ↑ energy ↑ erectile function ↑ stamina, fertility, and semen quality	Contains more than sixty phytonutrients and thirty-one trace minerals; has been used for thousands of years as a food source and an herbal remedy for people and animals. Completely safe and highly nutritious, maca tuber can be given to infants, pregnant women, and people with

(continued)

Herbal Supplement	Source	Effects	Notes
			chronic medical conditions.
Muira puama	Native Brazilian shrub	↑ erectile function ↑ energy ↑ orgasm ↑ mental acuity and mood	A 1990 study presented at the First International Congress of Ethnopharmacology in Strasbourg, France, "validated muira puama's safety and effectiveness in improving libido and sexual function."[13] Test tube experiments with rat brain tissue indicate that muira puama may have potential benefits in treating age-related cognitive decline and Alzheimer's disease.[14]
Nettle root (or stinging nettle root)	Leafy plant grown in temperate regions	↑ levels of free testosterone ↑ libido ↓ prostate enlargement	May have benefits in preventing prostate cancer. Has been used to treat male pattern baldness.

For Men and Women: Natural Aphrodisiacs Turn Up the Heat		
Herbal Supplement	Effects	Notes and Cautions
L-arginine	↑ release of nitric oxide, stimulating more blood flow to genital area ↑ libido ↑ frequency of orgasm ↑ feelings of sexual satisfaction	Do not take if you have low blood pressure, heart disease, liver disease, diabetes, genital herpes, or cold sores.
Ginkgo	Helps those suffering from antidepressant-related sexual dysfunction ↑ arousal and strength of orgasm	Ginkgo may increase bleeding risk. Do not take if you have a bleeding disorder or are having surgery, including dental procedures.
Ginseng	↑ nitric oxide, thereby ↑ sexual function and strength of orgasm	May lower blood pressure. People with diabetes should consult their doctor before using.
Horny goat weed	↑ libido ↑ energy ↑ erectile function and fullness ↓ symptoms of menstrual discomfort	Do not take if you have liver or kidney disease.
Yohimbe	↑ libido ↑ sexual function ↓ depression Promote weight loss	

You are reading this book because you miss the sex life you had when you were younger. You now know what foods and supplements will help restore that surge; now it is time for you to *do something*. If you really want to reignite those sexual fireworks, you need to get off your buns and get moving.

10

Step 3: Get Moving to Get Grooving

With his full head of silver hair, a thirty-six-inch waist, and an irrepressible spring in his step, 74-year-old Angus could easily pass for a man twenty years younger, which very much frustrated his 52-year-old son, Doug.

"It's downright humiliating," Doug complained as he took another gulp of beer.

"What is that, Son?" Angus asked before cutting into a huge piece of Alaskan wild salmon and taking a bite. "What has got you so down?"

"You and your way with women." Doug sighed. "I had really been enjoying Lenore's company these past several weeks. She loves sports, so I thought taking her to a hockey game might be a perfect entrée to my suggesting we cuddle up to get warm later. But, oh no. We get to our stadium box last night, she takes one look at you, and for the rest of the night I might as well have been moldy cottage cheese."

"Well, Lenore was pretty and lively, but I wouldn't snake my own son," Angus replied as he chuckled. "Besides, I swam a little longer than usual yesterday afternoon, which meant Betty and I only had time for a quickie before the game. I had a date to stop by her place and make up for it later on."

"Dad, whether or not you already had a date is not the point," Doug said as he downed the last of his beer and motioned to the waitress to bring him another. "It's just so embarrassing that every woman I have dated since my divorce has dropped me the minute she laid eyes on you. And speaking of 'laid' . . . Are you telling me that you had sex not once but twice in the same night? I can hardly manage once a week." Doug groaned and put his head in his hands.

"Doug," Angus said, suddenly serious, "sit up and look at me. Your problem with women is all about you and your bad habits. If you want the women to sway your way and if you want to be up to the occasion when they do, you have got to take better care of yourself. Put down those nachos, tell our waitress to take back that second beer, get off your barn door–size rear end, and go get some exercise."

Exercise is the third natural and nonnegotiable component in our three-step approach to revitalizing your sex life. Regular exercise positively impacts your hormone levels, increases blood flow to your genitals, whittles away those pounds around your middle, shifts that stress off your shoulders, and gives you the confidence and energy you need to get naked and have a great time. Bottom line: If you want to groove, you've got to move.

Exercise Revs Up Hormones

A Special Health Report published by Harvard Medical School states, "Exercise affects nearly all the hormones your body produces." And the bottom line is that more exercise equals more of the hormones you need to want and enjoy more sex. Unfortunately, the data indicates that Americans are exercising less and less as they get older.

In 2002, a British research team led by Pat Kendall-Taylor found that men aged 55 to 65 who ran regularly were found to have higher levels of testosterone and human growth hormone (HGH) than their sedentary counterparts. Ten runners from local athletic clubs and ten healthy but inactive men from local social clubs were recruited. The hormone profiles of all twenty were assessed while at rest and while doing exercise. The average level of testosterone in the runners was 25 percent higher and HGH levels were four times as high as those of the nonexercisers.[1]

In a study conducted at Baylor University in Texas, men's testosterone levels were found to peak forty-eight hours after lifting weights.[2] And the evidence suggested that the harder you train, the more you increase your natural levels of testosterone. Here are a few other interesting facts about how weight lifting can boost testosterone levels:

- When lifting weights, choose multijoint exercises that work your large muscle groups such as squats, dead lifts, bench presses, and rows. Studies have shown that these exercises can increase testosterone more than single-joint, small muscle–group movements.
- Studies have found that lifting weights that only allow you to do about five repetitions produces the greatest increase in testosterone levels.

- Do at least three sets of each exercise. Research suggests that you will get more testosterone production by doing three sets than you will by doing only one or two sets of heavy weights.
- Be sure to get adequate rest. Research shows that overtraining can actually hurt testosterone levels. A study at the University of North Carolina showed that overtraining could reduce testosterone levels by as much as 40 percent. Give muscles one full day to recover.

In addition to increasing testosterone and HGH, exercise elevates endorphins. These natural opiates help block pain perception and improve mood. The runner's high is a classic example of exercise-stimulated endorphin release. Your sex drive and feelings of sexual pleasure also use an endorphin-release system. The more frequent and intense the endorphin releases, the easier it is for sexual arousal and pleasure in the future. Studies have shown that women who frequently exercise become aroused more quickly and are able to reach orgasm faster and more intensely.[3]

Exercise Stimulates Sexual Appetite and Response

Deirdre, who is 43, enjoys exercise and sex with her husband:

> Our sex life moved to a whole new plane of pleasure once we began exercising together. We take a brisk thirty- to forty-minute walk every night before dinner and then have so much more energy throughout the evening. A couple of nights per week, Daniel will tuck the kids in for the night while I prepare some kind of bedroom surprise. I'll dress up in new lingerie, have the room lit with candles, or draw a warm bath for two. Who knew that getting out and moving would give us so much more get-up-and-go for each other?

Deirdre's experience is not unusual. Researchers at Bentley College in Massachusetts found that women in their 40s who exercised three to four times a week engaged in sex more often (about seven times per month) and enjoyed it more than a sedentary group of peers.[4] Researchers at the University of Texas in Austin studied thirty-five women between the ages of 18 and 34. On two separate occasions, the women watched a short travel film followed by a brief X-rated movie. The first time, the women cycled vigorously for twenty minutes before sitting down to watch the programs; the second time, they didn't. Researchers calculated their sexual response using a device that measures blood flow to the genital tissue and discovered that the women's vaginal responses were 169 percent greater when they cycled.[5]

Similarly, a 2003 study published in the *Annals of Internal Medicine* of middle-aged, sedentary men found that after just one hour of exercise three times a week, the men demonstrated improved sexual function, more frequent sex and orgasms, and greater satisfaction.[6]

Finally, 60-plus-year-old men and women who exercise regularly report having the same amount of sex and sexual pleasure as people decades younger. One study examined the sexual frequency and satisfaction of swimmers aged 60 and found that they were the same as those twenty years younger.[7]

Exercise Improves Erectile Function

Frank, who is 53, was both delighted and amazed:

> I loved to run in my 20s and 30s, but between the kids and my
> job, I rationalized letting that time go as I got older. If I had
> known that running every day would help me get and keep a

hard-on, I would never have stopped. After only six weeks of running three to four miles five days a week, I am experiencing a big difference. When aroused, my penis is packing as full as it did fifteen to twenty years ago. Even better, it stays engorged long enough for me to satisfy both my wife and me. I've decided to start training for a marathon. Makes you wonder what Forest Gump's erections were like, doesn't it?

When it comes to choosing a diet, what is good for your heart is good for your genitals, and the same holds true for exercise. It helps keep your heart and arteries healthy so that they are able to pump blood throughout your body, including your genital area. In 2004, results of an Italian research study published in the *Journal of the American Medical Association* showed that out of 110 obese men, 30 percent who had previously suffered from ED had firm, sustainable erections after two years of regular exercise.[8]

Exercise and Your Sexual Self-Esteem

When you look in the mirror, do you like what you see? Now, take a peek when you get out of the shower. Are love handles, flabby thighs, a wider butt, or droopy boobies making you feel self-conscious about your sexual attractiveness? You may not be able to stop an economic recession or solve world hunger in a month or two, but if you exercise for eight weeks, you can begin to feel differently about your body. Consider Desiree's experience:

When I turned 50, my husband gave me a gift certificate for fifty sessions with a personal trainer. Also in the box was a black lace negligee. At first, I was offended. Then I realized that the negligee was a size 12 and not a size 2. I thought, maybe Samuel isn't telling me I am fat. Maybe he is trying to help me once again feel good enough about my body so that I will get out of mu-mus and flannel nightgowns. I decided to give it a try and started going to the gym three days a week. It has been only two months, but I am wearing sleeveless tops and dresses for the first time in years. And, while my jeans are still a size 12, I don't have to wear ones with elastic in the back. Oh, and did I mention how I look in that negligee? I think I look pretty darn good with it on, but Samuel says I look even better when it's off.

Improving your sexual self-esteem is another great reason to get up and be active. Multiple studies have shown that men and women who exercise regularly feel more comfortable baring their bellies and hopping into the sack. Seventy-one percent of women who reported their fitness level above average also rated their sexual desirability as above average.[9]

How Sexually Fit Are You?

Sex is a physical activity. If your goal is to have more fun romping between the sheets, a certain degree of sexual fitness is required. No matter if you have formerly been a committed couch potato or are currently a seasoned athlete, you can choose exercises to progressively improve your level of sexual fitness. The following questions should help you determine what you need to focus on right now. Those with an injury, heart disease, or another preexisting medical condition should first consult their physician. Also, consider working out with a trainer who will design an exercise regimen to accommodate your special concerns.

1. How strong is your core?

     You won't have great sex if three minutes into it you don't have the strength to hold that position or can't move "there" for fear of injury. By practicing exercises that promote core stabilization, you will be better able to control your body through different planes and movements. In addition, core stabilization has been shown to help older and/or less flexible people better control their body's movement through awkward or unusual movements to avoid strain or injury.

     Core strengthening involves your lower back, abdominals, and pelvic region. For a simple core strength program, you can begin with push-ups and crunches. Other exercises that develop core strength include exercises on a stability ball, work with medicine balls (weighing from a couple of pounds to 25 pounds) and wobble boards (a piece of training equipment used to improve balance), and Pilates exercise programs. One of my favorite core exercises is the plank:

   - Start by lying facedown on the ground or on an exercise mat. Place your elbows and forearms underneath your chest.
   - Prop yourself up to form a bridge, balancing on your toes and forearms.
   - Maintain a flat back and do not allow your hips to sag toward the ground or arch up.
   - Hold for as long as you can.

2. How long and hard can you go?

     You can't really go for the gusto if you're out of breath with physical exertion. And, on a more positive note, one of the wonderful aspects about sex for more mature adults is that a quick "wham-bam-thank-you-ma'am" is not as exciting as extended sessions of touching and teasing.

To build up stamina and endurance, you will need to do cardio exercises. Shoot for five days per week of doing something you enjoy for at least thirty or forty minutes: walking, running, swimming, dancing, or taking an aerobics class.

3. Can you move "there" with no pain and a minimal amount of fuss?

Flexibility will increase your ability and willingness to shift from the plain old missionary to some spicy new sex positions. We become less flexible as we get older due to certain changes that take place in our connective tissues. As we age, our bodies gradually dehydrate to some extent. It is believed that stretching stimulates the production or retention of lubricants between the connective tissue fibers, thus preventing the formation of adhesions. Hence, exercise can delay some of the loss of flexibility that occurs due to the aging process. Yoga is a wonderful way to increase flexibility. If you start a regular stretching practice on your own, consider the following guidelines:

- Warm up first. Warm muscles, tendons, and ligaments are more flexible and stretch more easily; stretching cold muscles can cause tears.
- Stretches should always be gradual and gentle.
- Hold each stretch in a static position for ten to twenty seconds, allowing the muscle to lengthen slowly.
- Do not bounce; bouncing actually causes muscle fibers to shorten, not lengthen.
- Stretch only to the point of resistance; if the stretch hurts, you're pushing too hard.

- Don't rush through the stretching routine; use it to prepare yourself mentally and physically for activity.

We guarantee that when you combine sexy-healthy eating with herbal supplements and regular exercise, you will not only feel sexier, you will also look it. Your commitment to more heart-pumping and limb-strengthening exercise has even greater benefits. Getting back in the mood and having the energy for more sex can improve your health and extend your life. Read on to find out how.

Part Four:

Hormone Health and Heaven at Any Age

You are now happily convinced that you no longer have to resign yourself to the inevitability of declining hormone levels and a deteriorating sex drive. Whether you choose BHRT, the three-step approach, or a combination of both, you have safe and natural options for restoring hormone balance and turning back your sexual clock. Chapter 11 offers more good news: Regular sex (with all safe-sex precautions) is a health bonus. The physiologic benefits include positive weight management and overall fitness, a stronger immune system, a reduced risk of heart disease and prostate cancer, and more.

More frequent and satisfying sex can be a shot in the arm for relationships gone stale. Chapter 12 offers time-proven techniques and fresh ideas for how to deepen the emotional and spiritual intimacy made available through enhanced physical connectedness.

11

Balanced Hormones and More Sex: Your New Fountain of Youth

Now that your hormone balance is restored, your weeks are increasingly punctuated by more frequent and enthusiastic sex. There's a bounce in your step and a twinkle in your eye. Keep it up and you will reap multiple bonuses. Your active sex life is going to make you healthier, buffer, younger looking, and prone to live longer . . . that is, as long as you keep it safe.

Sex Makes You Skinnier

In 1975, Abel and Analise were college sweethearts. Their romance waned, however, after they graduated and took jobs in different states. In 2005, they reconnected at a thirty-year class reunion. Analise had been widowed ten years earlier and Abel had been divorced for four years. Analise was amazed by Abel's still fit physique and embarrassed that her five-four frame had taken on an extra 30 pounds. Abel, however, didn't mind. He insisted that Analise was just as lovely as ever. A hot and heavy romance soon ensued.

For several months, the couple rendezvoused on weekends. Their short time together always left them emotionally elated, physically spent, and longing for more. Finally, Abel begged Analise to pack up her computer and continue her freelance graphic arts business from his home base. She agreed to give it a try for one month. Analise raved to me about the three-step plan:

> My marriage had always been fraught with tension, so I was nervous about moving in with Abel. A few weeks after unpacking my suitcase, however, I couldn't believe how much fun we were having. Abel had been on your three-step plan for more than a year, so I joined right in. I shopped, he cooked, we walked or swam five days a week, and best of all, our provocative conversations and titillating sexual adventures got better and better as the days flew by. At the end of the month, we were even more in love. Better yet, I was 16 pounds lighter with a waistline 4 inches smaller.
>
> I am thrilled about how my body has responded to my new love life. I have tried diets and exercise before with very little results. Who knew that sex was what I needed to finally whittle my middle away?

Sex is a fun, calorie-burning exercise. A steamy twenty minutes of lovemaking can burn up to 200 calories, about the same as fifteen minutes on a treadmill or elliptical machine. In addition to burning up those calories, certain sexual positions have a workout benefit.

Think of those pelvic tilts you did in Pilates and the plank or downward dog pose you tried in yoga class. Now consider how you might put those moves to work in your bedroom. Ah-ha! Movements and muscular contractions during intercourse work muscles of the pelvis, thighs, buttocks, arms, and chest. *Men's Health* magazine has gone so far as to call the bed the single greatest piece of exercise equipment ever invented.[1] The opportunity to combine sensual delight with moves that tone your tummy, trim your buns, and strengthen your core should be splendid motivation for spending more time in the sack.

Sex Is Good for Your Heart

You've just had a half hour of steamy, hot sex. Your pulse rate is up and you feel your blood pumping as if you have just run three miles. Your heart is benefiting from more than love.

In 1997, a group of British researchers tracked the health of 918 men between the ages of 45 and 59 for ten years. During the study, 150 of the men died. When the researchers ran a statistical analysis to see whether there was a connection between sexual activity and the risk of death, they found something surprising. The risk of death from all causes was halved in men who reported the highest frequency of orgasm, compared to men with the least sexual activity. Mostly, there was a reduction in the number of deaths associated with heart disease.[2]

Recently, when Randy and I were presenting at a health conference, I noticed this lovely couple sitting in the front row holding hands. They looked to be in their early to mid-50s. When we shared data supporting our premise that great sex promotes good health, I saw the gentleman wipe away tears. When our talk concluded, the couple came forward and introduced themselves as Barry and Diane.

"Dr. Randolph, I only wish I could have heard this talk five or ten years ago," said Barry. "I was so busy traveling and growing my business that I put my love for Diane on the back burner for years. God knows how her feminine sexual esteem took a beating during all those times I would come home and barely look at her while I emptied one suitcase and packed another. Despite my neglect, Diane never stopped loving me. Three years ago, when I had a heart attack, this wonderful woman never left my side. Now it's too late. As much as I want to make love to my beautiful wife, I am afraid my heart can't take it."

"Barry," Randy said, "that may or may not be true. In general, sex puts the same amount of pressure on your heart as a brisk twenty-minute walk, and an orgasm is the equivalent of a walk up the stairs. Statistics suggest that only 1 percent of heart attacks are triggered by sexual activity. And, observing how taken you are with Diane, this next statistic should be added encouragement: It is estimated that 75 percent of deaths that occur during sexual intercourse are in men who are having extramarital relations with women much younger than themselves. What has your cardiologist advised?"

"Before today, I have been too embarrassed to talk about it," Barry confessed. "But not anymore. You have given me new hope. I am going to call my doctor tomorrow and see what he says."

Like Barry, many people who have suffered a heart attack give up sex out of fear that the activity might trigger another cardiovascular event. The risk is low. In fact, many physicians encourage an active sex life because it provides cardiovascular exercise. If you have had a heart attack or have a heart condition, talk to your doctor about what he or she recommends.

Sex Boosts Your Immune System

According to a 2007 Fox News Report, sexually active people take fewer sick days and are less prone to catch colds or the flu. The reason is that frequent sex has been proven to boost the immune system. Medical researchers at Wilkes University in Wilkes-Barre, Pennsylvania, found that individuals having sex once or twice a week had a 30 percent higher level of an antibody called immunoglobulin A (IgA), whose function is to heighten immune system response.

Sex Eases Pain and Takes the Edge Off

Oxytocin is a hormone that is released by the brain during touching, kissing, cuddling, and intercourse, with a spike at orgasm. Not only does touch stimulate the production of oxytocin, but oxytocin promotes a desire to be touched more: It's a feedback loop with wonderful implications.

Immediately before orgasm, levels of oxytocin surge to five times their normal level. This, in turn, releases endorphins and corticosteroids, which act as analgesics to help reduce or alleviate pain. This physiologic response has been shown to offer pain relief for those suffering from migraines, chronic back or neck pain, and menstrual cramps.

Sex is also a super stress-buster. Researchers in Scotland studied how the sexual activity of twenty-four women and twenty-two men impacted their blood pressure response to stressful situations, such as speaking in public or doing verbal arithmetic. Those who had intercourse had lower blood pressure response than those who engaged in other sexual activities or who had no sex at all.[3] New research has revealed that when women are stressed out, they release more oxytocin than adrenaline, thus triggering the need for interpersonal interaction.[4]

Other studies show that the oxytocin released during sex promotes a good night's sleep. Tired of tossing and turning for hours on end? Try taking a tumble with your lover instead.

Sex Protects the Prostate

A 2004 study published in the *Journal of the American Medical Association* reported that frequent intercourse or masturbation resulting in ejaculation helps to protect men against prostate cancer. The study followed thirty thousand men over an eight-year period. At the start of the study, men of all ages filled in a history of their ejaculation frequency and completed additional questionnaires every two years. Men who had more than twelve ejaculations per month were found to have a significantly reduced incidence of prostate cancer.[5] These results backed the findings of a smaller Australian study published in *New Scientist* in 2008.[6]

Sex Makes You Feel Closer and Act Kinder

A few weeks before Christmas, I got an interesting call from one of our patients:

> Genie, Brad and I are both on BHRT, following your diet, and exercising more. Our sex life has improved dramatically; whereas we were having sex maybe once a month, we now have sex three to four times a week. But that is not why I called. Something weird is happening to Brad's personality. Usually at Christmas he

grudgingly dóles out a few dollars for presents for the kids and insists that we only exchange cards with other family members and our friends. This year, however, he went to the mall and bought treats for my parents, his cousins, and even our neighbor's dog. I love the change, but I'm worried. Could all this sex be making his brain soft?

Chuckling, I told her that I was pretty sure Brad's brain was fine. But the sex was changing him. At a cellular level, a hormone released during sex was making his heart more generous.

An interesting study in the November 2008 issue of *Psychological Science* by Christian Unkelbach, Adam Guastella, and Joseph Forgas followed a group of men given either a dose of oxytocin or a placebo. The men took a recognition test for positive and negative words related to sex, relationships, other positive emotions, and words unrelated to positive emotions. The study found that men who had been given oxytocin more readily accessed positive words related to sex and relationships. The findings suggest that oxytocin release makes it easier for men to act in a positive and loving way toward their sexual partners.[7] This study was done only with men, but similar kinds of results have been obtained with women.[8]

Don't wait for New Year's resolutions. If a sexual surplus will make you a kinder, more loving, and generous partner, why not get on the stick today?

Medical Issues

Illness or disability, such as stroke, diabetes, cancer, arthritis, or mental illness, can affect your sex life, but it doesn't mean that you have to shut down that facet of your life for good. Talk to your doctor about your degree of sexual fitness and readiness. And if you struggle with the feeling that your body has betrayed you, first remind yourself that you are still here and thus have the potential to experience pleasure. If depression or fears don't abate, seek the help of a trained counselor. Finally, consider a shift in your health not as an end game but as a challenge for discovering different, rather than dampened, ways to channel and express your innate sensuality.

Better Safe than Sorry

Great sex can do your body good, but first make sure you are having safe sex. Think you are too old to be concerned about the risk of sexually transmitted diseases (STDs)? You are not. Consider what happened to Quinn:

> I was devastated when my wife of forty-five years died of cancer. I grieved deeply for more than three years, then one day it dawned on me: I was only 64 years old, I could live two to three more decades, and those years were looking pretty lonely. I knew my wife wouldn't have wanted me to stay in the house moping around. She would have told me to get out and get on with my life.
>
> I started dating a 59-year-old divorcée named Faye who I had known for more than twenty years. She worked for my dentist and we attended the same church. When we became physically intimate, I knew Faye was long past the years when pregnancy was a worry, so it never occurred to me to wear a condom. Two years later, a routine blood test revealed that I had contracted HIV.

A 2008 study published in the journal *Sexually Transmitted Infections* reported that STD rates had more than doubled among adults 45 and older.[9] Like Quinn, many older adults believe that condoms are unnecessary because pregnancy is not an issue. They are uninformed about the increasing prevalence of STDs for sexually active men and women in their age group.

Physicians may overlook the importance of sex education for their older patients because of time constraints or the misconception that sex is not a factor once patients are past a certain age. Lack of screening for sexual diseases in the over-60 crowd increases the risk of an STD going undiagnosed for years, which can lead to serious health consequences.

If you are considering having sex with a new partner— whether it is with someone you have known for decades or someone you just met via the Internet—engage in safe sex. Before you are intimate with a new partner, you and your potential lover should exchange current blood work results indicating a clean bill of health. Without the blood work, never, ever have sex without a condom.

Feeling uncomfortable about how to request this life insurance? Take a hint from my friend Shirley, a 53-year-old divorcée who told the "perfect match" she had met online, "Let's throw a bedroom party on the date we share the results of our lab work. You chill the champagne, and I'll bring the lingerie and a new set of black silk king-sized sheets." According to her, once the champagne popped, they never had time to put on those new sexy sheets.

No matter what your age, if you have had unprotected sex, you should ask your primary care physician to screen you for HIV. If you are a woman, you should also be screened for cervical cancer, which can be caused by the sexually transmitted virus

HPV. Regular cervical screening via a pap smear is an effective way to catch early cancerous changes before they start to cause problems.

First, you learned how to safely restore youthful hormone levels and revitalize your sex life. Now you understand how the benefits of regular sexual activity extend far beyond more fun in the sack. A buffer, healthier, happier, and more sensual you is more in the mood than ever before. Now it's time to work on the emotional side of things.

12

New Emotional Highs for Old and New Relationships

Here's a news flash: Women and men think differently. Okay, okay . . . you knew that already, but did you know that hormones have a lot to do with the difference between the male and female minds? The predominantly male hormone testosterone, or "Mr. T," is linked to characteristics like aggressiveness, self-assertiveness, competitiveness, independence, and goal accomplishment. Estrogen and progesterone, the hormones more prevalent in women, are the hormones most associated with nesting and nurturing feelings as well as the desire for connectedness.

When Mr. T is in charge, men tend to regard sex as an event or something to be accomplished. What's the point in romance and foreplay? Let's get right to it, most men think, even if they don't say it. Many men feel the act of sex is the same thing as intimacy. In fact, when men need emotional bonding and intimacy, they will seek out sex from their partner.

Women, however, have a different point of view. Because of

estrogen and progesterone's influence on the female mind and emotions, a woman regards sex as much more than a trigger for physical release. At its best, sex for a woman is a convergence of intellectual, emotional, spiritual, and physical stimulation. Rather than seek out sex to feel more intimate, women want to experience feelings of intimacy before they have sex. "I want to feel as if we are in tune with each other. I can't just flip a switch, get in the mood, and hop into bed," a woman might say, or, "Doesn't he get that there is more to life than lust?"

With such different perspectives, it is a wonder that relationships ever work. But they do. And however bad, good, or humdrum your relationship feels now, it can get better. Feeling in the mood again is just the beginning. The following five tips will help women and men get more of everything they want.

Tip 1: Put It on Your Calendar

Remember when you were in your teens and you and your boy/girlfriend could hardly stand to sit through an entire movie before leaping up, out, and into the backseat of the car? Those were the days when nothing (other than curfews, parents, and a possible shotgun) got in the way of your wanting to touch, taste, and enjoy. Today, there are easily a dozen things standing in your way: jobs, children, aging parents, laundry, bills, yard work . . . you get the drift. No wonder it is so easy for sex to fall behind on your list of to-do's.

Our first (and possibly the most important) tip: Make time for sex. Literally. Put it on your calendar. Make a date with your partner. Keep that time slot sacred and nonnegotiable. And allow at least one hour.

"Why an hour if we can accomplish our mission in fifteen or

twenty minutes?" you might ask (and "you" are probably a man). Because great sex is an experience, not just an event. Making a date for sex certainly paid off for Betsy and Phil:

> When you first suggested that Phil and I put time for sex on our calendars, I felt relief. I juggle a demanding job and the care of a mother with dementia, as well as my household responsibilities. Time is my most precious commodity, and being organized down to the minute is how I stay sane. So when Phil would spontaneously try to initiate sex in the morning, all I could think about was how behind I would be for the rest of the day if we did it. Our sexual pleasure was greatly diminished because when I gave in, I was always watching the clock. If I put him off, he felt rejected. It was a no-win situation.
>
> Scheduling time for sex was our salvation. I literally started writing "important personal meeting" on my calendar, and just as I would for a business meeting, I set aside time beforehand to prepare. Washing my hair, trying on lingerie, and picking out mood music allowed me the time to mentally switch off all my other to-do's and focus on how best to share this special time with my husband. I planned how to get Phil to tune into me and us rather than simply hopping to it. When I started "going to bed" in my mind long before he and I were in the bedroom, the emotional and mental foreplay allowed for sweeter connections as we warmed up to each other and a mutually satisfying joining later.

Phil appreciates the scheduling, too:

> I was uneasy about the idea of putting time for sex on my weekly calendar, but after the first time, I realized that Betsy was more

present when we made love than I had felt her in years. On our first date for sex, I came to bed loaded and ready for action, but Betsy curled up next to me and suggested we talk first. "Talk about what?" I asked. "How nervous we were the first time we went to bed" she replied.

Before you knew it we were laughing and telling stories about good times together. At some point, Betsy reached over and began to massage my penis. I drew back at first because—with all the talking and laughing—I had stopped focusing on having sex and, consequently, lost my erection. Betsy gently but firmly kept her hand in place and continued the massage all the while reminiscing about the time we had sex on the beach. When I was fully aroused again, we had sex and it was wonderful for me, but I worried that it had taken me too long to come. "Was that too much work for you?" I asked. "Are you kidding?" Betsy replied. "I felt so emotionally entwined with you today that I wanted the experience to last as long as possible." Now, our scheduled trysts are the part of my week that I most look forward to.

Tip 2: Be a Kind and Patient Listener

Women are typically tagged "the talkers," but both women and men need to be seen and *heard* in a healthy relationship. Open communication about your emotional needs and listening closely to your partner's feelings are building blocks for the ability to please and be pleased emotionally and sexually. According to relationship and intimacy coach Richard Nicastro, "When in-depth listening is lost, the fallout is significant: One or both partners might feel marginalized; there may be increased conflict, lingering resentments, emotional withdrawal, deep despair, or a loss of hope."

If an underlying hormonal imbalance is causing you to be irritable, depressed, or anxious, your ability to be a kind and patient listener will be compromised and your relationship will suffer. Tend to this first. This book has already given you a toolbox of things to help. Commit to listening with greater intention and attention, and experience the seductive power of new, or renewed, intimacy. You might be surprised at the difference ten minutes and one heartfelt question can make. Consider the experience of the following couple.

Harrison, a soft-spoken man in his late 50s, leaned forward anxiously:

> Marilyn says she has lost interest in having sex with me because I have no idea who she really is. That is absolutely crazy. We have been married for twenty-two years and have raised a son together. She says she wants a trial separation and then possibly a divorce if some form of intimacy is not restored in our relationship. That is exactly why I want to have sex . . . to give us back some of the intimacy our relationship is missing.

Looking at Marilyn, I waited for her to speak:

> We haven't had a real conversation in years. I am always talking over the television or trying to get Harrison's attention away from his computer screen. Your bioidentical hormones and three-step plan not only helped me get through menopause, they helped me reclaim my body, mind, and emotions. I may be older, but I feel more whole than ever. Having sex with someone who doesn't know anything about what I am feeling or thinking would be giving away an important part of myself and getting nothing in return. I am no longer willing to pay that price.

My turn to talk:

Harrison, for the next three weeks I want you to try spending ten minutes a day simply listening to Marilyn. Ask her how she is feeling about your relationship, your son's direction in life, the two of you getting older, or simply her opinion on a controversial topic in the daily news. Be engaged and make eye contact. Watch the need to interrupt or look bored. You need to turn off the TV or cell phone, close your mouth, open your ears, and really pay attention. If Marilyn brings up an issue or problem, try not to offer any quick fix-it solutions. And during these three weeks, I am asking you not to put any pressure on Marilyn to have sex.

Harrison didn't look too happy, but he agreed to give it a try. A month later, the couple came back to see me. This time they walked in holding hands. Marilyn told me:

At first, our conversations were quite stilted. Then one day, Harrison asked me if I ever thought about the baby I miscarried before I became pregnant with our son. I burst into tears, because there is not a day that goes by that I don't wonder about the woman our daughter would have grown into. He cried, too. I had no idea that the loss of that baby was still on his heart as well.

After that, our conversations began to move into previously uncharted emotional waters. We first talked about other sadness or regrets we had from our youth. One day, when I confided how I wished I had taken ballet as a child, Harrison told me he had always thought of me as a ballerina. I asked why, and he answered, "When you climax, you throw your head back and arch your neck just like those beautiful ballerinas we saw years ago on stage in New York." I was completely taken aback that he viewed me with such romantic eyes.

Harrison sat quietly until I turned his way:

I honestly feel years younger than I did a month ago. Learning something new about my wife almost every day has been excit-ing. Each conversation has brought us closer. And Marilyn was right: I didn't really know her. I had no idea how the girl I had married had blossomed into such a smart, savvy, and stimulating woman.

"How has it been for you to forego sex during this time?" I asked. But it was Marilyn, not Harrison, who answered.

"Genie, you said to abstain for three weeks," she said as she squeezed Harrison's hand and inched closer on the sofa. "This is week number four."

Tip 3: Find a New Passion to Share

A big reason relationships go stale over time is that when nothing feels novel, boredom can set in. One of the best ways to stir up new feelings of excitement in the bedroom is to discover another new hobby or interest to share as a couple. Finding a new sport you both enjoy is one great option, and we have discussed how more exercise will benefit your sex life, but I also suggest you do something beyond the physical. Round out your relationship by finding a new interest that jazzes you both up intellectually and/ or emotionally. Sandra and Tony certainly benefited from ex-panding their horizons:

When Tony started having weekly testosterone injections, he was soon ready to have sex at a moment's notice. I went along with it, but the sex just wasn't that satisfying. Tony sensed my boredom and asked if I wanted him to try a new technique or for us to experiment with some kind of sex toy. I told him it really wasn't the sex; it was just that I felt like we had drifted apart mentally and emotionally. I was sorry after I said it, because he wanted to "fix it" and I didn't have any idea how we could. The truth was that it wasn't just the sex, hanging out with Tony was no longer stimulating or fun in any way.

You see, we talked a lot, but we shared little. Our conversations centered on our children, chores around the house, or financial decisions. When it came to sharing feelings, I turned to my girlfriends. For intellectual stimulation, I relied on TV talk shows and my book club. Then two things happened. First, Tony saw a video called *The Secret* and got real excited about the metaphysical power of positive thoughts. For the first time ever, we started having discussions about spirituality and the purpose of our lives. Then, for Christmas, my parents enrolled us in an Italian food cooking class and told us they would keep the kids when we went. I never thought Tony would go, but to my surprise he was gung-ho. Now, we pore over recipe books together, tend to a new herb garden, and enjoy entertaining our friends with special new dishes. What is most wonderful is that I feel like I have fallen in love with a new man. Our sex life feels fresh and adventurous. I am more into it—and him—than ever before.

Tip 4: Believe Your Body Is Good Enough to Share

In Chapter I, my sister Sheila voiced her concern about "unclothing a body with some road miles on it." Sheila is not alone. Researchers have found that people with a poor body image are more likely to avoid sexual activities and struggle with sexual functioning. The problem is more prevalent in women. Statistics show that for those over 40 years old, 33 percent of men indicate that body dissatisfaction negatively influences their sex life, and a whopping 70 percent of women report that their feelings of sexuality are depressed by concerns about their weight or body shape.

BHRT and/or the three-step plan will help you trim down and tone up, but nothing, not even the nips and tucks of plastic surgery, will fully restore your body to the effortless magnificence of its youth. Still, regardless of your current size or shape, I want you to look in the mirror and see something beautiful. Seriously. Your body has carried you this far, so it deserves to be a source of celebration. I encourage you to regard any wear and tear on the outside as a badge of what you have gone through to be so much better on the inside. As Marianne Williamson says, "While you may be feeling a bit depressed that you are no longer young, you should be ecstatic that you are no longer clueless."

While my pep talk may offer encouragement, my guess is that it won't allay all your concerns about stripping down if you are not (yet) in the shape that you want to be in. The following hints will give you more confidence:

- Get clean. Good hygiene will enhance your attractiveness. And you will smell better. Try incorporating a shared bath, shower, or gentle genital washcloth wipe-down into your sexual warm-up rituals.

"I love it when Maurice and I take a bath together," says 61-year-old Edna. "He either starts sudsing my toes or my ears and moves slowly toward my more erogenous zones from there. When it is my turn to lather him up, I have him sit with his back against my chest. With my arms around him, I run my hands from his chest to his abs and then down a little further."

- Moisturize your skin and take care of your nails. Dry, flaky skin and yellowish, jagged nails are for old people long past their prime. That most definitely should not be you. Exfoliate rough patches of skin, like elbows and knees, then rub on moisturizing lotions or creams. Even better, let your partner rub them on for you. Trim and clean your nails; they will look better and you won't risk scratching your partner. Put on some nail polish if you like, but be sure to allow enough time for it to dry. Scheduling a professional manicure and pedicure could be a fun way to start your date night.

- Practice good posture. No one looks good when their body slumps forward, causing fat or loose skin to fall into rolls or folds. Stand up straight, stretch out long when lying down, and engage your torso, or core, as you move into your favorite sexual positions.

- Dress for sex and experiment with lingerie. If you are a woman whose body is pear shaped—your hips, buttocks, and thighs are where you carry your extra weight—choose a low-rise or bikini-cut panty to emphasize your smaller waist. A baby-doll nightie can provide some masking of your hip area, or try a long nightgown with a low-cut bodice to draw attention above your waist.

If your body is shaped more like an apple—most of your weight is carried around your middle—teddies with very high sides can paint your figure in flattering lines. Corsets, bustiers, and waist-cinching garments will also create the illusion of a more hourglass shape.

Men should also try new undergarments to show off their best parts. First and foremost, keep them clean. Men's boxers and briefs continue to be the most popular styles. Consider branching out from plain white to colored silk. The more adventurous man might try a bikini, or speedo look, or even a leather thong.

"When we have sex, my wife typically leaves on her short nightie and I keep on my silk boxers," says 48-year-old Nathan. "She is not as self-conscious, making her more willing to move around into different positions, and I find the feel of silk mixed with skin to be exceptionally titillating."

Tip 5: Ask for What You Want

In the fall of 2008, a group of our patients asked me to be the lunchtime speaker for their senior citizen's bridge club. I was given forty-five minutes, so I alloted thirty minutes for an instructional lecture on hormones and libido, ten minutes to take their questions, and five minutes for me to use the audience as an ad-hoc focus group. "I hope I have shared enough medical information that you are encouraged that you can have great sex no matter your age. Now I have a favor," I told the crowd as my assistant passed out pens and index cards. "Please share with me your advice for making sex past 50 or 60 better than sex at 20 or 30. Don't worry about signing your name."

The following excerpts are from their responses. See if a common theme jumps out at you as it quickly did for me:

For thirty years, I silently endured my ex-husband's wham-bam-thank-you-ma'am approach to sex. When we divorced and I eventually started dating, I determined that if I was going to have sex with a man again, it was time for me to stop acting like a shrinking violet and ask for the kind of sex I had always dreamed about. What has been most wonderful is that I soon discovered that the more specific my requests, the more it turns on my partner.

I love that as my husband has aged, it takes him longer to climax. Rather than spend those extra minutes doing the same old thing, we have developed a repertoire of ways to please each other and take turns asking for what we want.

When I was a 20-something boy, I could get an erection looking at the curve of a soup spoon. Now, to get firm, I require more manual or oral stimulation. The necessity of asking for what I need has opened a whole new realm of experiences for me and my wife. She is much more comfortable putting me on hold and saying, "My turn now." The swapping of requests has taken our lovemaking to exciting new heights.

Taking a note from my friends here, I will now give you my bottom line: Restored hormone balance will increase your libido and improve sexual function, but hormones alone won't guarantee you sexual satisfaction.

Thank goodness, you are more self-aware, self-confident, and experienced than you were at 20 or 30. If you want more, different, or better sex, now is not the age for you to waste time fumbling around. Talk to your mate or lover. Tell him or her what feels good and what doesn't. Risk sharing your sexual fantasies and desires. Ask for the sexual pleasure you have been waiting your whole life to experience. Now is your time to generously give and joyfully receive.

APPENDIX A:
A WEEK OF
SEXY-HEALTHY EATING

In Chapter 7, you learned how nutrition plays a vital role in boosting and balancing the hormones you need to enjoy a quality sex life. Now we pull all the diet details together in a weekly menu of meals that will rev you up and tantalize your taste buds. These delicious daily feasts include a parade of succulent fruits and vegetables paired with delectable seafood or savory meat dishes. The food combinations are intended to spark your imagination, stir your libido, and fuel more energy for between-the-sheets delights. Even better, preparing these dishes with passion in mind will set the mood for a night or day of lovemaking. And, *wow*, sexy-healthy eating helps those extra pounds around your middle start to melt away. Get ready to start licking your lips and thinking of love!

Your Grocery List

The following grocery list is intended to stock you up with everything the two of you will need for a week of sexy-healthy eating. Check your cabinets and refrigerator first to see what ingredients you might have. Some items, such as the spices, are an investment that will last for months. Again, when at all possible, choose organic.

Veggies
10 tomatoes
1 head cauliflower
1½ lb. turnip greens
2 avocados
3 lb. fresh spinach
2 lb. carrots
1 bunch celery
7 onions
2 bunches green onions
1 red pepper
1 yellow pepper
1 zuchini
2 yellow squash
16 oz. spring salad mix
1 cucumber
8 oz. shallots
1 jalapeño pepper
10 Brussels sprouts
fresh oregano
fresh basil

Fruits
4 grapefruits
14 lemons
1 pint blueberries
1 pint strawberries
4 apples
2 pears
2 mangoes
4 bananas
1 16 oz. can frozen
    orange juice
    concentrate
1 lb. fresh cherries
2 peaches

Protein
8 6-oz. chicken breasts
½ lb. sliced turkey
    breast
1 6-oz. can tuna,
    packed in water
1 8-oz. can sardines,
    packed in oil
3 lb. fresh sardines
1½ lb. smoked salmon
1½ lb. ground turkey
2 lb. calves liver
1 lb. turkey bacon
4–6 lb. turkey breast
2 lb. flank steak
2½ dozen raw oysters
2 dozen large shrimp
1 lb. salmon fillets

Dairy
1 dozen eggs
2 8-oz. containers of
    plain low-fat yogurt
1 32-oz. carton low-
    fat soy milk

Dry Goods
1 24-oz. loaf whole-
    grain or whole-
    wheat bread
1 5.25-oz. box sesame
    seed melba toast

Other
16 oz. extra-virgin
    olive oil
6 cloves garlic or
    1 8-oz. jar
    minced garlic

Dairy

2 8-oz. containers vanilla or lemon yogurt

16 oz. low-fat cottage cheese

8 oz. feta cheese

4 oz. goat cheese

½ gallon low-fat or skim milk

16 oz. grated Parmesan cheese

Dry Goods

⅓ lb. each walnuts, cashews, almonds, pistachio nuts, pine nuts, and hazelnuts

3 8-oz. cans mandarin oranges in juice

1 8-oz. box raisins

1 5.6-oz. box couscous

1 lb. whole-wheat corkscrew pasta

18 oz carton/container slow-cooking oatmeal

1 15-oz. can kidney beans

1 15-oz. can green beans

2 15-oz. cans garbanzo beans

4 14.75–15-oz. cans diced tomatoes

1 4-oz. jar capers

1 4-oz. can sliced black olives

1 17-oz. package whole-grain hamburger buns

32 oz. vegetable broth

16 oz. chicken broth

8 oz. dried cranberries

1 4-oz. can green chilis

1 jar apricot preserves

8 oz. brown rice

1 box whole-grain dry cereal

Other

1 container milled flaxseeds

1 bunch fresh rosemary

1 bunch fresh parsley

Poppyseeds

Dried ginger

1 1-lb. jar honey

Rice wine vinegar

Balsamic vinegar

Cayenne pepper

Red pepper flakes

Tobasco

Garlic powder

Curry powder

Paprika

Bay leaves

Black pepper

Dried parsley

Dried thyme

Dried Italian seasoning

1 56-oz. bag dark chocolate Hershey kisses (can freeze to keep fresh)

2 bottles red wine

4–6 chocolate-dipped strawberries from your favorite sweet shop (wait to purchase these on day 6)

A Week of Menus

Remember that my approach is to satisfy you nutritionally while stimulating you sexually. There is no calorie counting—tune in and trust your body to tell you when you are hungry and when you are full. Do your best to keep to a 6-ounce serving of protein and ½ cup of cooked whole grains, but when it comes to the veggies, feel free to scoop up a second helping. Healthy snacking wards off feelings of deprivation. Sexy-healthy eating is a "more" experience.

For a tantalizing prelude, work fresh herbs with your hands, then let your partner catch the scent when he or she kisses your fingers, or slowly feed your partner a taste of what is cooking. Set the table with flowers and candles. If you have kids still at home, pack them off to a sleepover for a night, throw a blanket on the floor, put on your pajamas (or take them off), and have a bedroom picnic. Take your time to savor each bite as you share a meal. Rediscover how erotic the art of eating can be.

Note: Recipes follow for menu items marked with an asterisk (*).

Day 1

Breakfast
Scrambled eggs
½ Broiled Grapefruit*
Whole-wheat toast
Hot water with lemon and a dash of cayenne pepper

Snack
A few walnuts
Water

Lunch

Canned tuna tossed with fresh spinach and a small can of
mandarin oranges packed in water (not syrup) and drained,
garnished with slivered almonds

Steamed asparagus tossed in lemon juice, olive oil, and flaxseeds

Sesame seed melba toast

Water

Snack

Blueberries stirred in plain, vanilla, or lemon low-fat yogurt

Water

Dinner

Marinated and Grilled Chicken Breasts*

Mashed Cauliflower*

Tangy Turnip Greens*

Whole-grain bread

1 4-oz. glass of red wine (if desired)

Water

Day 2

Breakfast

Smiley Toast*

Low-fat soy milk, flavor of your choice

Hot water with lemon and a dash of cayenne pepper

Snack

Orange or tangerine

Water

Lunch

Turkey, Broccoli, and Cashew Roll-ups*

Couscous with Tomatoes and Parmesan*

Water

Snack

Apple and hazelnuts

Water

Dinner

Spicy Pasta with Fresh Sardines*

Fresh Spinach Salad Tossed with Feta and Red Peppers*

1 4-oz. glass of red wine (if desired)

Water

Day 3

Breakfast

Smoked salmon

Slow-cooked oatmeal with berries

Hot water with lemon and a dash of cayenne pepper

Snack

Celery and carrot sticks

Water

Lunch

Open-Faced Turkey Burger*

Three-Bean Salad*

Cottage cheese tossed with grapefruit or orange slices and
    flaxseeds

Water

Snack

Pear and almonds or pistachio nuts

Water

Dinner

Savory Calves Liver with Fresh Rosemary and Turkey Bacon*

Brown rice

Steamed spinach tossed with extra-virgin olive oil and lemon juice

   and topped with sliced boiled egg

1 4-oz. glass of red wine (if desired)

Water

Day 4

Breakfast

Egg in a Nest*

Berries

Hot water with lemon and a dash of cayenne pepper

Snack

Grapefruit tossed in low-fat yogurt

Water

Lunch

Vegetable Barley Soup*

Dreamy Fruit Salad*

Water

Snack

2 Hershey kisses and macadamia nuts

Water

Dinner

Vegetable-Stuffed Flank Steak*

Broiled Tomatoes with Garlic*

Brown rice

1 4-oz. glass of red wine (if desired)

Water

Day 5

Breakfast

Whole-grain dry cereal with banana or berries and low-fat or
   skim milk

Water with lemon

Snack

Almonds or walnuts

Water

Lunch

Sardine Salad*

Apple

Sesame seed melba toast

Water

Snack

Orange Smoothie with Flaxseeds*

Water

Dinner

Roast Turkey Breast with Sage and Garlic*

Steamed asparagus tossed with extra-virgin olive oil, lemon juice,
   and crushed almonds

Sautéed yellow squash and zucchini

1 4-oz. glass of red wine (if desired)

Water

Day 6

Breakfast

Turkey bacon

Spinach, Asparagus, and Feta Omelet*

Orange or tangerine

Hot water with lemon and a dash of cayenne pepper

Snack

Whole-grain toast with preserves

Water

Lunch

Turkey Walnut Salad with Cranberries on Mixed Greens*

Baked Apples with Ginger and Cinnamon*

Water

Snack

Almonds or walnuts

Water

Dinner

Raw Oyster Appetizer with Spicy Dipping Sauce*

Shrimp and Oyster Soulful Supper*

Green salad with avocado and tomato dressed with extra-virgin
    olive oil and lemon juice

1 4-oz. glass of red wine (if desired)

Water

Day 7

Breakfast

Smoked salmon

Citrus Ambrosia*

Whole-wheat or whole-grain toast, dry

Hot water with lemon and a dash of cayenne pepper

Snack

Almonds or walnuts

Water

Lunch

Spicy Chicken and Green Chili Soup*

Spinach salad with mandarin oranges and boiled egg with honey-
    lime dressing

Snack

Chocolate-dipped strawberries (2–3 each)

Soy milk

Water

Dinner

Apricot Honey-Ginger Salmon*

Brussels sprouts

Fresh peaches and cottage cheese

1 4-oz. glass red wine (if desired)

Water

Recipes

Day 1

BROILED GRAPEFRUIT

Serves 2

1 grapefruit

1 teaspoon ground ginger

1 tablespoon honey

1. Preheat the broiler.

2. Cut the grapefruit in half and use a small serrated knife to cut out the sections. Spoon the sections and juice into a bowl. Scrape out all of the remaining thick skin and pulp and discard. Spoon the sections from the bowl back into the halves. This is best done one-half at a time.

3. Sprinkle the ginger and drizzle the honey over the top of each grapefruit half. Place the halves on a baking sheet.

4. Broil for 3 to 5 minutes, until the honey begins to bubble.

MARINATED AND GRILLED CHICKEN BREASTS

Serves 2

½ cup lemon juice

1 tablespoon extra-virgin olive oil

2 6-ounce skinless, boneless chicken breast halves

1 teaspoon chopped fresh rosemary

1 teaspoon chopped fresh oregano

1 teaspoon chopped fresh basil

Ground black pepper to taste

1. Preheat an outdoor grill for medium-high and lightly oil the grater.
2. Combine the lemon juice and olive oil, dip the chicken in this mixture, then sprinkle with the rosemary, oregano, basil, and pepper.
3. Grill the chicken for 10 to 15 minutes per side, or until no longer pink and the juices run clear.

MASHED CAULIFLOWER

Serves 4–6

1 large head cauliflower, cut into florets
3 cups chicken broth
2 tablespoons minced garlic
¼ cup grated Parmesan cheese
Salt, pepper, and a dab of butter to taste

1. Bring the cauliflower, chicken broth, and garlic to a boil in a pot over high heat. Reduce the heat to medium, cover, and simmer for 10 minutes. Uncover the pot and increase the heat to medium-high. Allow the cauliflower to simmer until soft and the cooking liquid has reduced by half, about 10 minutes.
2. Remove the cauliflower from the heat and add the Parmesan cheese. Mash with a potato masher until smooth, then season to taste with salt and pepper. Add just a dab of butter if you must.

TANGY TURNIP GREENS

Serves 4

2 tablespoons extra-virgin olive oil
1 bunch green onions, chopped
1 teaspoon red pepper flakes

1½ pounds turnip greens, washed, chopped, stems removed

1 cup chicken broth

2 tablespoons rice wine vinegar

1. Heat the olive oil in a pot over medium heat.

2. Add the green onions and red pepper flakes. Sauté until tender and fragrant.

3. Add the turnip greens and chicken broth and cook until wilted, 2 to 3 minutes. Drain the greens in a collander.

4. Add the rice wine vinegar, toss, and serve immediately.

Day 2

SMILEY TOAST

Serves 2

1 tablespoon sesame seed butter (may substitute almond or peanut butter)

2 slices whole-grain or whole-wheat bread, toasted

½ banana

2 dozen raisins

1. Spread the sesame seed butter on the warm toast.

2. Use the banana slices to make eyes.

3. Arrange the raisins in a semicircle like a smile.

TURKEY, BROCCOLI, AND CASHEW ROLL-UPS

Serves 2

½ pound thinly sliced roast turkey breast

1 tablespoon honey

1 teaspoon lemon juice

½ teaspoon grated fresh ginger

½ cup finely chopped steamed broccoli

¼ cup crushed cashews

1. On a cutting board or on wax paper, separate the turkey slices into two
    piles.
2. In a small bowl, whisk together the honey, lemon juice, and ginger,
    then add the broccoli and cashews.
3. Spread the mixture on the turkey slices, roll up, and secure with
    toothpicks.

COUSCOUS WITH TOMATOES AND PARMESAN

Serves 4–6

1 tablespoon extra-virgin olive oil

1 large sweet onion, sliced

1 14.5-ounce can diced tomatoes

2 tablespoons balsamic vinegar

1 cup couscous

1 cup vegetable stock

¼ cup grated Parmesan cheese

Red pepper flakes to taste

1. Heat the olive oil in a grill pan over high heat. When the pan is very hot,
    add the onions. Press down occasionally to get grill lines across them.
    Turn as needed to prevent burning. Cook for about 15 minutes, or until
    evenly browned and cooked through.
2. Add the tomatoes and balsamic vinegar. Simmer for a few
    minutes.

3. Place the couscous in a heatproof medium bowl. Bring the vegetable stock to a boil in a pot over high heat, pour it over the couscous, and stir with a fork. Keep stirring the couscous to prevent sticking. It only takes 2 to 3 minutes to become soft.

4. Stir in the tomato–onion mixture.

5. Top with the Parmesan cheese and sprinkle with red pepper flakes as desired.

SPICY PASTA WITH FRESH SARDINES

Serves 4

3 pounds whole fresh sardines, boned, heads removed

1 cup extra-virgin olive oil

2 medium onions, diced

1 28-ounce can diced tomatoes

1 tablespoon dried fennel

1 tablespoon dried celery seed

½ teaspoon powdered saffron

3 tablespoons pine nuts

1 pound whole-wheat corkscrew pasta

1. Chop the sardines, reserving a few whole ones for garnishing.

2. Pour the olive oil in a skillet and sauté the onions and whole sardines over medium heat. Once the onions are caramelized (3 to 5 minutes), remove the whole sardines and reserve.

3. Add the tomatoes, fennel, celery seed, saffron, and pine nuts. Bring the sauce to a boil, then lower to simmer.

4. Add the chopped sardines and cook until they break into pieces, merging into the sauce, approximately 10 to 15 minutes.

5. Prepare the pasta according to the package directions.

6. Drain the cooked pasta and toss with the sauce. Let sit for a minute or two for the flavors of the sauce to soak in.

7. Garnish with the whole sardines.

FRESH SPINACH SALAD TOSSED WITH FETA AND RED PEPPERS

Serves 2

1½ cups fresh spinach, stems removed, well washed

¼ cup low-fat feta cheese

1 red pepper, sliced

Extra-virgin olive oil

Balsamic vinegar

1. In a bowl, toss the spinach, feta cheese, and red pepper together.

2. Dress with olive oil and balsamic vinegar to taste.

Day 3

OPEN-FACED TURKEY BURGER

Serves 4

1½ pounds ground turkey

1 cup frozen chopped spinach, thawed and drained

2 crumbled tablespoons goat cheese

2 tablespoons chopped black olives

Dash of cayenne pepper (optional)

2 whole-grain hamburger buns

1. Preheat the broiler.

2. In a medium bowl, mix together the ground turkey, spinach, goat cheese, olives, and cayenne pepper. Form the mixture into 4 patties.

3. Arrange the patties on a broiler pan, and broil for 15 minutes, turning once, or until done. Meanwhile, boil a pot of water. Place the buns in a colander and set on top of the pot of water, being careful not to let water in. The steam will soften the buns in 2 or 3 minutes.

4. Serve each turkey burger on top of a bun half.

THREE-BEAN SALAD

Serves 6

1 15-ounce can garbanzo beans (chickpeas), drained and rinsed

1 15-ounce can kidney beans, drained and rinsed

1 15-ounce can green beans, drained and rinsed

4 green onions, chopped

1 stalk celery, diced

1 cup steamed broccoli florets

1 red pepper, chopped

1 yellow pepper, chopped

½ cup cider vinegar

¼ cup extra-virgin olive oil

1 tablespoon honey

½ teaspoon dry mustard

¼ teaspoon garlic powder

¼ teaspoon ground black pepper

¼ teaspoon onion powder (optional)

¼ teaspoon cayenne pepper (optional)

¼ cup pine nuts

1. In a bowl, gently mix together the garbanzo beans, kidney beans, green beans, green onions, celery, broccoli florets, and peppers.

2. In a separate bowl, whisk together the vinegar, olive oil, honey,

mustard, garlic powder, black pepper, onion powder, and cayenne
pepper.

3.   Pour the cider vinegar–olive oil dressing over the salad, and toss gently
to coat.

4.   Cover, refrigerate at least 2 hours, add the pine nuts, and gently toss
before serving.

SAVORY CALVES LIVER WITH FRESH ROSEMARY AND TURKEY BACON

Serves 6

2 pounds calves liver, cut into 6 pieces

1 egg, lightly beaten

1 cup low-fat or skim milk

6 slices turkey bacon

1 large onion, chopped

3 tablespoons extra-virgin olive oil

½ cup whole-wheat bread crumbs

2 tablespoons chopped fresh rosemary

1 tablespoon red wine

1.   In a large baking dish, soak the liver in a mixture of the egg and milk for
20 to 30 minutes, then pat dry with a paper towel.

2.   Cook the turkey bacon in a skillet over medium-high heat until crisp.
Drain on paper towels. Then crumble into a bowl.

3.   Sauté the onion in 1 tablespoon olive oil in the skillet until brown and
tender. Transfer to the bowl with the turkey bacon and mix together.

4.   In a large plastic resealable bag, toss the liver with the bread crumbs
and 2 tablespoons fresh rosemary until it is fully coated.

5.   Add the remaining 2 tablespoons olive oil and the red wine to the

skillet, add the liver, and heat for 3 to 4 minutes on high heat on each side. Then simmer until most of the liquid evaporates.

6. Serve the liver topped with the onion and crumbled bacon mixture.

Day 4

EGG IN A NEST

Serves 2

2 slices whole-grain bread

Extra-virgin olive oil

2 eggs

2 tablespoons grated Parmesan cheese

Red pepper flakes to taste

1. Turn a small glass upside down to cut a circle out of each bread slice.
2. Lightly coat a skillet with olive oil, place the bread slices in the skillet, and break an egg into each hole.
3. Cook on medium heat, turning once until the eggs are the desired firmness.
4. Remove from the skillet and garnish with the Parmesan cheese and red pepper flakes.

VEGETABLE BARLEY SOUP

Serves 8

2 quarts vegetable broth

1 cup uncooked barley

2 large carrots, chopped

2 stalks celery, chopped

1 14.5-ounce can diced tomatoes with juice

1 zucchini, chopped

1 15-ounce can garbanzo beans, drained and rinsed

1 onion, chopped

3 bay leaves

1 teaspoon garlic powder

1 teaspoon salt

½ teaspoon ground black pepper

1 teaspoon dried parsley

1 teaspoon curry powder

1 teaspoon paprika

1 teaspoon Tabasco (optional)

1. Pour the vegetable broth into a large pot. Add the barley, carrots, celery, tomatoes, zucchini, garbanzo beans, onions, and bay leaves.
2. Season with the garlic powder, salt, pepper, parsley, curry powder, paprika, and Tabasco.
3. Bring to a boil, then cover and simmer over medium-low heat, stirring occasionally, for at least 1 hour.

DREAMY FRUIT SALAD

Serves 4

¼ cup lemon juice

2 teaspoons grated lemon zest

1 cup plain yogurt

1 tablespoon honey

1½ teaspoons poppyseeds

1 11-ounce can mandarin orange segments, drained

2 mangoes, peeled and sliced

1 banana, sliced

½ cup golden raisins

Spinach leaves

1. For the dressing, combine the lemon juice, lemon zest, yogurt, honey, and poppyseeds in a small bowl.
2. In a large bowl, combine the orange segments, mangoes, banana slices, and raisins. Add the dressing and toss to coat. Cover and refrigerate for 2 hours. Serve in a spinach-lined bowl.

VEGETABLE-STUFFED FLANK STEAK

Serves 6

2 pounds flank steak

½ cup red wine vinegar

3 cloves garlic, finely chopped

2 teaspoons dried thyme

1 cup fresh spinach

4 large carrots, boiled and cut in ½-inch pieces

1 cup sun-dried tomatoes soaked in red wine

1 small onion, thinly sliced

3 teaspoons red pepper flakes

2 tablespoons extra-virgin olive oil

1½ cups beef broth

1. Arrange the steak on a cutting board so that the long side is parallel to you. Using a long knife, butterfly the steak to within ½ inch of the far edge so that it opens like a book.
2. Pound the steak with a mallet until about ¼ inch thick. Transfer to a baking dish, poke holes in the meat, and sprinkle with the red wine vinegar, garlic, and thyme. Cover and marinate overnight.

3. Preheat the oven to 375° F. Put the meat on the cutting board and top with a layer of the spinach, carrots, sun-dried tomatoes, and onions. Sprinkle evenly with the red pepper flakes.

4. Starting with the edge closest to you, roll the meat forward to form a tight cylinder. Using kitchen twine, tie the meat at 1-inch intervals.

5. Heat the olive oil in a large, deep skillet or Dutch oven and sear the meat on all sides over high heat until brown.

6. Pour in the beef broth, then add enough water to reach about one-third of the way up the sides of the meat.

7. Cover, transfer to the oven, and bake until tender, approximately 2 hours.

8. Remove the meat and place on a clean cutting board. Let stand 10 minutes before slicing. Spoon a tablespoon of the beef broth mixture over the meat before serving.

BROILED TOMATOES WITH GARLIC

Serves 4

4 large tomatoes

1 tablespoon crushed garlic

1 tablespoon dried Italian seasoning

2 tablespoons extra-virgin olive oil

2 tablespoons grated Parmesan cheese

1. Preheat the broiler.

2. Slice the top of each tomato, then slice into the tomatoes from both sides so that they open up like a flower. Place the tomatoes on a baking sheet.

3. Sprinkle the tomatoes with the garlic, Italian seasoning, and olive oil, making sure that some of each goes into their center.

4. Top with the Parmesan cheese.
5. Broil until bubbly, 3 to 5 minutes.

Day 5

SARDINE SALAD

Serves 4

2 teaspoons red wine vinegar

2 teaspoons lemon juice

2 tablespoons plain yogurt

Ground black pepper to taste

2 large avocados, halved, pitted, and peeled

2 4-ounce tins of sardines packed in oil

12 pimiento-stuffed green olives, chopped

3 tablespoons finely chopped cucumber

3 tablespoons finely chopped celery

4 green onions, finely chopped

2 tablespoons chopped capers

1 cup mixed spring greens

1. To make the dressing, whisk together the red wine vinegar, lemon juice, and yogurt.
2. In a medium bowl, combine the avocados, sardines, olives, cucumbers, celery, onions, and capers.
3. Pour the dressing over the salad and toss. Chill for 4 to 8 hours. Serve on a bed of mixed spring greens.

ORANGE SMOOTHIE WITH FLAXSEEDS

Serves 4

1 banana

1 6-ounce can frozen orange juice concentrate

2 cups vanilla soy milk

1 teaspoon ground ginger

2 tablespoons milled flaxseeds

1. Place the banana, orange juice concentrate, soy milk, and ginger in a blender. Process until the ingredients are blended and smooth.
2. Stir in the flaxseeds and serve.

ROAST TURKEY BREAST WITH SAGE AND GARLIC

Serves 6–8

4–6 pounds turkey breast

¼ cup lemon juice

1 tablespoon honey

1 teaspoon ground black pepper

¼ cup extra-virgin olive oil

3 cloves garlic

1 cup fresh sage leaves or 3 tablespoons dried sage

3 onions, thinly sliced

6 ounces shallots, thinly sliced

2 carrots, cut in 2-inch pieces

¼ cup chopped fresh parsley

1. Preheat the oven to 475° F.
2. Pierce the turkey breast with a fork and place in a greased baking dish.

3. In a bowl, combine the lemon juice, honey, pepper, olive oil, garlic, and sage. Pour this mixture over the turkey breast.

4. Arrange the onions, shallots, and carrots around the turkey.

5. Roast for 15 minutes, then reduce the oven temperature to 400° F.

6. Cook until done, about 1 hour.

7. Let the turkey rest about 10 minutes, slice, arrange on a platter with the vegetables, and garnish with the parsley.

Day 6

SPINACH, ASPARAGUS, AND FETA OMELET

Serves 2

1 egg

3 egg whites

¼ teaspoon red pepper flakes

¼ teaspoon minced garlic

⅛ teaspoon ground black pepper

½ cup chopped asparagus spears

2 teaspoons extra-virgin olive oil

1 cup torn fresh spinach washed and dried

3 tablespoons crumbled tomato and basil feta cheese

1. In a small bowl, beat together the egg and egg whites. Add the red pepper flakes, garlic, and pepper. Mix well and set aside.

2. In a skillet, sauté the asparagus in the olive oil over medium-high heat for 2 to 3 minutes, or until tender. Add the spinach; cook and stir until the spinach is wilted. Add the egg mixture and top with the feta cheese.

3.   As the eggs set, lift the edges with a spatula, letting the uncooked portion flow underneath. Cut the omelet into wedges to serve.

TURKEY WALNUT SALAD WITH CRANBERRIES ON MIXED GREENS

Serves 4

2 cups diced cooked turkey

½ cup dried cranberries

1 cup diced celery

½ cup chopped walnuts

¼ cup low-fat plain yogurt

1 teaspoon honey

¼ teaspoon ground ginger

¼ teaspoon ground black pepper

1 cup mixed spring greens

1.   In a large bowl, toss together the turkey, cranberries, celery, and walnuts.

2.   In a small bowl, whisk together the yogurt, honey, ginger, and pepper. Spoon the dressing over the salad mixture and toss until well blended. Serve over a bed of mixed greens.

BAKED APPLES WITH GINGER AND CINNAMON

Serves 2

2 tablespoons chopped walnuts

¼ teaspoon grated orange zest

¼ teaspoon ground ginger

1 tablespoon butter, melted

1 tablespoon honey

2 tart apples

1. Preheat the oven to 350° F.

2. Combine the walnuts, orange zest, ginger, butter, and honey in a small bowl.

3. Core the apples and place in an ungreased 1½-quart baking dish.

4. Pour the butter–honey mixture over and around the apples. Bake for 30 to 35 minutes, until the apples are tender. Let stand 15 minutes before serving.

SPICY DIPPING SAUCE (FOR RAW OYSTERS)

Sufficient for 2 dozen oysters

⅓ cup extra-virgin olive oil

⅓ cup rice wine vinegar

1 teaspoon chili garlic sauce (in grocer's Asian food section)

1. Put the olive oil, rice wine vinegar, and chili garlic sauce in a bottle with a lid on it and shake.

2. Pour into small ramekins for dipping.

SHRIMP AND OYSTER SOULFUL SUPPER

Serves 4

¼ cup chopped green onions

1 onion, chopped

1 jalapeño pepper, seeded and chopped

2 tablespoons chopped garlic

2 tablespoons extra-virgin olive oil

1 teaspoon dried thyme

½ teaspoon cayenne pepper

½ cup chicken broth

1 20-ounce can chopped tomatoes

1 cup brown rice

2 dozen large shrimp, peeled and deveined

1½ dozen shucked raw oysters

1. In a large pot over medium-high heat, sauté the onions, jalapeño pepper, and garlic in the olive oil. Add the thyme and cayenne pepper. Cook until tender, about 5 minutes.

2. Stir in the chicken broth, canned tomatoes, and rice. Bring to a boil, then reduce the heat to simmer until the rice is cooked through, about 20 minutes.

3. Stir in the shrimp. Cook until the shrimp turn pink, about 5 minutes. Add the oysters and stir for 1 minute.

Day 7

CITRUS AMBROSIA

Serves 2 to 3

1 11-ounce can mandarin oranges, drained

1 pink grapefruit (or grapefruit sections in a jar, packed in juice, not syrup), cut into ½-inch pieces

2 tangerines, cut into ½-inch pieces

1 cup fresh cherries, pitted and halved

⅛ cup slivered almonds

1. Toss all the ingredients together and chill for 1 hour.

2. Serve in a martini glass, just for fun.

SPICY CHICKEN AND GREEN CHILI SOUP

Serves 4

1 large onion, chopped

2 cloves garlic, minced

1 tablespoon extra-virgin olive oil

4 skinless, boneless chicken breasts, cut into bite size pieces

2 cups chicken broth

2 teaspoons chopped canned green chili peppers

1 8-ounce can diced tomatoes

¼ cup chopped fresh cilantro

1. In a large pot or Dutch oven, cook the onions and garlic in the olive oil over medium heat until tender, about 4 minutes.
2. Add the chicken, chicken broth, chili peppers, and tomatoes.
3. Bring to a boil, then reduce the heat and simmer for 15 minutes. Garnish with the cilantro.

APRICOT HONEY-GINGER SALMON

Serves 2

2 teaspoons extra-virgin olive oil

1 tablespoon honey

2 teaspoons grated fresh ginger

1 pound salmon fillets

1 tablespoon apricot preserves

1. Preheat the oven to 350° F.
2. In a small bowl, combine the olive oil, honey, and ginger.

3. Place the salmon fillets in a greased baking dish, pierce the flesh all over with a fork, and pour the olive oil–honey mixture over the salmon.

4. Top with the apricot preserves and bake for 15 to 20 minutes, or until the salmon flakes easily with a fork.

APPENDIX B: RESOURCES

The contact information listed in this section was current as of the publication of this book.

Hormone Health

The Natural Hormone Institute

When Randy and I cofounded the Natural Hormone Institute in 2003, we had two goals in mind. The first was to create a vehicle to educate both the medical community and the health care consumer about the safety and efficacy of bioidentical hormone therapies and herbal remedies to support overall hormone health. Our second goal was to formalize a business entity to make our over-the-counter bioidentical progesterone cream and other signature herbal remedies and supplements more widely available and commit a percentage of Web site profits to support medical research in the field of bioidentical hormone replacement.

For more information regarding bioidentical hormone replacement, to discuss scheduling a personal consultation, or to purchase the products recommended in this book, go to our interactive Web site www.hormonewell.com, or contact our office by calling (866) NAT-MEDS/628-6337.

Over-the-Counter Progesterone Creams

You can purchase bioidentical progesterone creams in most health food stores. The good news is that they are available. The bad news is that some products are better than others. There is no regulatory body that oversees the production or standardization of product manufacturing for so-called natural products. What this means to the average consumer is that there is great variation among the many over-the-counter progesterone creams on the market today.

While we cannot reveal our exact formula for Dr. Randolph's Natural Balance Cream, I can outline some of the critical variables that define its excellence and efficacy:

- Dr. Randolph's Natural Balance Cream is a bioidentical formulation of progesterone. The molecules of progesterone suspended in the cream have exactly the same molecular structure as those produced by the human body. The body recognizes, receives, and utilizes these molecules. The parent molecule for progesterone comes from a substance known as diosgenin, which is found in soy or Mexican wild yam. Many products on the market today that contain soy or Mexican wild yam claim to be natural progesterones; however, until the diosgenin is converted from its original molecular structure, the body will not recognize it. Consequently, soy or Mexican wild yam in the raw state will not generate the same clinical response.

- Dr. Randolph's Natural Balance Cream contains the maximum concentration of bioidentical progesterone that can be mixed in an over-the-counter product. Some other creams have a little progesterone in their mix but not enough to generate a consistent and positive patient response.

- The progesterone we use in our formula meets the United States Pharmacopoeia gold standards for quality and purity. In addition, we require the lab that produces Dr. Randolph's Natural Balance Cream to compound the product under strict guidelines approved by the National Association of Compounding Pharmacists. This is not required by law, so not all product manufacturers go to the trouble or expense.

- The progesterone molecule in our cream is encased within a liposomal delivery system. This is critical, because as the many layers of the oily globule of liposome melt away, the hormones are dispersed continuously through the skin for up to twelve hours. Hormonal balance is restored, and women and men have continuous relief of their symptoms throughout the day. In contrast, other over-the-counter progesterone creams are not formulated for sustained release. Since the progesterone in these other over-the-counter creams is immediately absorbed through the skin, the result is a quick spike in progesterone levels and only a temporary relief of symptoms.

There are several other over-the-counter progesterone creams that we have reviewed for quality and truth in advertising. These include:

Arbonne International
PhytoProlief and Prolief Natural Balancing Creams
P.O. Box 2488

Laguna Hills, California 92654

(800) ARBONNE or www.arbonne.com

Emerita

Pro-Gest Progesterone Cream

621 S.W. Alder, Suite 900

Portland, Oregon 97205-3627

(800) 648-8211 or www.emerita.com

Health and Science Research Institute

Serenity for Women Progesterone Cream

661 Beville Rd., Suite 101

Daytona Beach, Florida 32119

(888) 222-1415 or www.health-science.com

HM Enterprises

Happy PMS

2622 Bailey Dr.

Norcross, Georgia 30071

(800) 742-4773 or www.hmenterprises.com

Life-flo Health Care Products

Progestacare Cream

8146 N. 23rd Ave, Suite E

Phoenix, Arizona 85021

(888) 999-7440 or www.sheld.com/lifeflo

Products of Nature

Natural Woman Progesterone Cream

54 Danbury Rd.

Ridgefield, Connecticut 06877

(800) 665-5952 or www.pronature.com

Restored Balance, Inc.

Restored Balance PMS/Menopausal Progesterone Cream

42 Meadowbridge Dr., S.W.

Cartersville, Georgia 30120

(800) 865-7499 or www.restoredbalanceusa.com

There are many other progesterone creams on the market today that we have not reviewed, and they may also contain bioidentical progesterone. If you have doubts or concerns regarding a bioidentical progesterone product, call the company and ask how many milligrams of progesterone per ounce the cream contains.

Over-the-Counter Bioidentical Estriol

Estriol is one of the three principal estrogens that are produced by the body. Research has shown that estriol promotes breast health, bone density, heart health, and postmenopausal urinary tract health. It also helps protect against multiple sclerosis and vaginal dryness. Dr. Randolph's Natural Estro-Fem Cream is a bioidentical formulation of estriol. This means that the molecules of estriol suspended in the cream have exactly the same molecular structure as those produced by the human body. The estriol molecule in Dr. Randolph's Natural Estro-Fem Cream is incased within a liposomal delivery system. This is critical, because as the many layers of the oily globule of liposome melt away like a snowball, the hormones are dispersed continuously through the skin for up to twelve hours.

Herbal Products Boost Libido and Sexual Vitality

Age-related decline in testosterone production is a problem for both sexes. Bioidentical testosterone is not available in an over-the-counter formulation so, if this is your choice for boosting a lagging libido and improving sexual performance, you will need to see a doctor and get a prescription. You do, however, have another safe and effective option.

Drawing on Randy's original training in pharmacognosy (plant-based medicine) and my decades of research into centuries-old herbal approaches to improving sexual desire, performance, and pleasure, we developed an all-natural signature sexual vitality product line that jump-starts your libido, increases energy, improves blood flow, and enhances feelings of tactile stimulation. Men now have a choice that is safer, and as effective and less expensive that Viagra or Cialis. These herbal products also help women re-ignite passion and restore feelings of sensual enjoyment and pleasure. Our sexual vitality product line is available online at www.hormonewell.com.

When You Need a Prescription

Our experience has been that close to 80 percent of women and men can safely and effectively self-treat symptoms of hormone imbalance with over-the-counter bioidentical and herbal formulations. When symptoms persist, however, your body is signaling that you need something more. It may be time for a personalized hormone level profile possibly followed by a prescription.

Prior to seeing a physician, it is possible for you to obtain a personal hormone level profile so you know exactly what is going on inside your body at a cellular level. On our Web site, we offer two options: ZRT Laboratory and MyMedLab, Inc. For many years, Randy has used ZRT Laboratory (www.salivatest.com) for accurate measurement of a broad array of hormones and detection of hormone imbalance via saliva and blood spot testing. Dr. David Zava, founder of ZRT Laboratory, is also the coauthor with John R. Lee, M.D., of *What Your Doctor May Not Tell You About Breast Cancer.* Collecting a saliva sample can be conveniently accomplished at home and then mailed to the lab. More recently, Randy has worked with MyMedLab (www.mymedlab.com) to develop a signature profile for blood analysis of hormone levels. These are available direct to consumers without a doctor's visit or appointment at more than two thousand collection sites across the United States. We also offer telephone consultations to interpret results and recommend next steps; however, our medical professionals cannot legally prescribe BHRT—or any medication—until they have seen a patient in person.

With your hormone level profile in hand, a knowledgeable physician can then determine your recommended prescription for BHRT. In our medical practice, we compound each prescription based on the individual's need. As described in Chapter 5, compounding pharmacies customize individual prescriptions and can vary by dosage strength, choices of fillers (for example lactose-free), options for delivery including creams, drops, tablets, capsules, etc... The advantage of a compounded formulation of BHRT is that it can be titrated (increased or decreased) based on individual response.

Some physicians, however, prefer to prescribe pharmaceutically-manufactured bioidentical hormones because they have a higher comfort level treating their patients with standardized doses. Pharmaceutically-manufactured bioidentical hormone therapy drugs can also be a great option for women and men who want a more traditional prescription accompanied by a package insert. Though these products do not allow for individualized variations, they are FDA approved and are typically reimburse-able by insurance companies. Options include:

Bioidentical Estradiol

Note: due to estrogens propensity to promote cell growth, you should never take/use any form of estrogen—even bioidentical—without also taking/using bioidentical progesterone.

Divigel: Gel formulation available in multiple dosage strengths; Upsher-Smith Laboratories, Inc.; www.divigelus.com.

Estrasorb: Soy-based lotion typically prescribed as treatment for hot flashes; Grace Pharmaceuticals; www.estrasorb.com.

EstroGel: Gel formulation prescribed to help manage hot flashes, night sweats, and vaginal dryness and itching; Ascend Therapeutics; www.estrogel.com.

Evamist: A once-daily spray prescribed for moderate to severe hot flashes; Ther-Rx; www.evamist.com.

Estrace: Vaginal cream typically prescribed for vaginal atrophy, dryness, and post-menopausal urinary infections. Contract Pharmaceuticals, Ltd; www.rxlist.com/estrace-drug.htm.

Bioidentical Progesterone

Prochieve 8%: Vaginal gel typically prescribed to optimize progesterone levels to support therapy for infertility. Columbia Laboratories; www.prochieve8.com.

Prochieve 4%: Vaginal gel typically prescribed to treat progesterone deficiency and symptoms of estrogen dominance before, during, and after menopause. Manufactured by Fleet Laboratories, Ltd., marketed by ASCEND Therapeutics; www.prochieve4.com.

Prometrium: Capsules typically prescribed to treat progesterone deficiency and symptoms of estrogen dominance before, during, and after menopause. Solvay Pharmaceuticals; www.prometrium.com.

Bioidentical Testosterone

Androgel: A bioidentical testosterone gel packaged in a pump or packet for daily use. Solvay Pharmaceuticals; www.androgel.com.

Testopel: The only implantable bioidentical testosterone pellet currently on the market. A physician inserts Testopel pellets under the skin in a 10-minute, in-office procedure done once every 3 to 6 months. Some men prefer the convenience of a testosterone therapy that is effective for months versus a product requiring daily application or even compounded weekly or bi-weekly injections. Randy and I particularly love the following quote from Oliver Wendell Holmes featured on the testopel Web site: *"Men do not quit playing because they grow old, they grow old because they quit playing."* Slate Pharmaceuticals; www.testopel.com.

Locating a Physician

If you are looking for a physician in your area who is knowledgeable about BHRT, contact your local compounding pharmacist. If you need help finding a compounding pharmacy in your area, contact one of these two organizations:

International Academy of Compounding Pharmacists (IACP)
P.O. Box 1365
Sugar Land, Texas 77487
Phone (281) 933-8400

Fax (281) 495-0602

www.iacprx.org

IACP was established in 1991 as Professionals and Patients for Customized Care (P2C2). In 1996, P2C2 changed its name to IACP in an effort to broaden its scope and recognize changes in the profession. Today, IACP has more than eighteen hundred members internationally, serving pharmacists, physicians, students, and patients.

Professional Compounding Centers of America (PCCA)

9901 South Wilcrest Dr.

Houston, Texas 77099

Phone (877) 798-3224

Fax (877) 765-1422

www.pccarx.com

PCCA provides independent pharmacists with a complete support system for compounding unique dosage forms. Founded in 1981, PCCA has more than three thousand pharmacist members throughout the United States, Canada, Australia, Europe, and New Zealand. On average, PCCA's consulting department answers more than five hundred calls per day, providing members with comprehensive technical support.

Sexy-Healthy Foods and Vitamins

Grocery Stores

Founded in 1980 as one small store in Austin, Texas, Whole Foods Market is now the world's leading retailer of natural and organic foods, with 197 stores in North America and the United Kingdom. To find a Whole Foods Market near you, go to www .wholefoodsmarket.com.

Web Sites

Many people initially complain that buying organic is too expensive. Organic foods can be pricey if you just shop in your supermarket, but you probably have a lot more choices for organic foods in your community than you realize. All it takes is a little research.

To find a source of organic foods near you or to order online, check out the following Web sites: www.organicfoods.com, www .organicconsumer.org, www.eatwell.com, and www.diamond organics.com. Also, local farmer's markets can be a great source for organic foods, often at lower prices than you will pay in the supermarket or health food store.

Vitamins and Supplements

When Randy opened his first Natural Medicine Store, he stocked the shelves with natural products from a variety of manufacturers. It was not long before the difference in his patients' and customers' responses signaled that not all product manufacturers could be trusted. According to a recent survey of nearly one thousand supplements conducted by ConsumerLab.com, a product certification company, one out of four supplements has quality problems, such as contamination or a failure to include an ingredient listed on the label.

As Randy became aware of the discrepancy between manufacturers, he drew on his professional training and experience as a compounding pharmacist to establish criteria that would ensure that products in his shop, and now on our Web site, are safe and effective.

His criterion for our private-label products is simple and nonnegotiable: *quality and truth in labeling.* For our own private-label line, as well as for other natural health product lines that we carry, we require stringent manufacturing guidelines that include:

- Raw materials testing
- Potency testing
- Product traceability
- Purity testing
- Product freshness
- Microbiology testing

The bottom line is truth in packaging. People have the right to know what they are putting in their body, and they deserve to get the amount of active ingredient they are paying for.

To order Dr. Randolph's products online, go to www .hormonewell.com.

Life Extension is a very reliable source for vitamins and supplements. This company's manufacturing standards ensure exceptional purity and quality. In addition to its natural product offerings, Life Extension publishes a fantastic monthly magazine. For more information on Life Extension, go to www.lef.org or call (800) 226-2370.

Whole Grains

Just because a bread, cereal, or pasta product is brown in color, don't assume that it is a whole-grain product. Check the ingredients list for the words *whole grain* or *whole wheat* to decide whether the product is made from a whole grain. Some foods are made from a mixture of whole and refined grains.

Some grain products contain significant amounts of bran, which provides fiber and is important for health. However, products with added bran or bran alone (e.g., oat bran) are not necessarily whole-grain products.

On their Web site, www.wholegrainlife.com, General Mills offers excellent information regarding "What Is a Whole Grain?" and "How to Find a Whole-Grain Product." General Mills products are readily available in every grocery store across the nation.

Kashi (www.kashi.com) is one of my favorite whole-grain brands. I particularly love the company's logo: "7 Grains on a Mission." We stock Kashi products in both of our Natural Medicine Stores. They are also available in the health food or organic food aisle in grocery stores.

Another brand to check out is Food for Life (www.food forlife.com). I am a huge fan of its organic sprouted whole-grain pastas and breads. We stock Food for Life products in our Natural Medicine Stores. To find out where you can buy them, check out the Web site's built-in store finder.

Weight Loss

Body weight and sexual self-esteem tend to go hand-in-hand. When you feel good in your body, you are more inclined to share it with someone you care about. When you feel fat, the tendency is to cover yourself up and crawl under the covers to hide. Losing the weight you want and keeping it off for good helps keep you in the mood for life.

When our book *From Belly Fat to Belly Flat* was released in early

2008, Randy and I were thrilled to finally get the word out about the link between hormone imbalance (specifically estrogen dominance) and abdominal weight gain. We soon heard from throngs of women and men who excitedly told us, *"I have a waist again!"* *"Those stubborn pounds around my tummy, butt, hips, and thighs are finally gone."* And, best of all, *"I am back into my skinny jeans and I look great."* But, unfortunately, we also had some readers who told us *"I lost some pounds but not all the weight I want or need to."* Or, *"Those pounds came off but three months later I had gained it all back. I am so tired of my weight yo-yo'ing. What am I doing wrong?"*

We knew from experience that our Belly Flat Plan included the essential keys for sustained weight loss: hormone balancing, a sound nutritional program, vitamins and supplements, and exercise and lifestyle recommendations. Nevertheless, we fully understood why it is not a panacea for all.

Weight gain is not simply a physiologic issue. Emotional eating—eating to soothe/suppress negative feelings of anxiety, sadness, anger, frustration, or low self esteem—can sabotage weight-loss efforts. Persons who have repeatedly tried in vain to lose weight, or who have experienced years or yo-yo weight loss/weight gain, often need extra help to safely get and keep those pounds off. This help may come in the form of counseling, a more regimented and supervised nutritional program, a monitored food diary, and ongoing opportunities for individual encouragement and group support. We committed to extend our reach beyond our book to better help more people lose their unwanted pounds once and for all.

In 2009, our Natural Hormone Institute entered into a strategic partnership with Metabolic Research Center. We identified this organization as our partner of choice because not only do they offer a medically-based, nutritionally-balanced approach to weight loss but, more important to our perspective, their program uniquely integrates hormone balancing with holistic principles and positive life-management skills. More than simply helping individuals make better meal choices, we witnessed how Metabolic Research Center's integrated philosophy helped long-suffering women and men finally overcome both hormone imbalance saboteurs and the emotional side of eating.

We are aware of no other weight-loss program on the market today that effectively incorporates all these essential variables to help you not only to lose weight quickly, safely, and effectively, but to keep it off for a lifetime. To learn more, or to find a Metabolic Research Center near you, go to www.emetabolic.com or call (800) 501–8090.

Organic Housecleaning Products

Remember that it is important to decrease your exposure to environmental estrogens, or xenoestrogens. I recommend using organic housecleaning products when at all possible. Two good sources for online purchasing are www.heathersnaturals.com and www.organiccleaning.com.

Safe Cosmetics

I urge you to make sure that your cosmetics are safe. Many are not. The Campaign for Safe Cosmetics is a coalition of public health, educational, religious, labor, women's, environmental, and consumer groups. The coalition's goal is to protect the health of consumers and workers by requiring the health and beauty industry to phase out the use of chemicals linked to cancer, birth defects, and other health problems, and replace them with safer alternatives.

The Safe Cosmetics Campaign began in 2002 with the release of a report, *Not Too Pretty: Phthalates, Beauty Products and the FDA*. For the report, environmental and public health groups contracted with a laboratory to test seventy-two name-brand, off-the-shelf beauty products for the presence of phthalates, a family of industrial chemicals linked to permanent birth defects in the male reproductive system.

You can find a listing on the Safe Cosmetics Campaign Web site, www.safecosmetics.org/companies/signers.cfm, of the companies that have pledged not to use chemicals in their products that are known or strongly suspected of causing cancer, mutation, or birth defects and to implement substitution plans that replace hazardous materials with safer alternatives in every market they serve.

Several major cosmetics companies, including OPI, Avon, Estee Lauder, L'Oreal, Revlon, Procter & Gamble, and Unilever, have thus far refused to sign the Compact for Safe Cosmetics.

The good news is that safe cosmetics are readily available. Just head to your nearest health food store or mall.

Recommended Reading

Books

Randy and I have written two other books, *From Hormone Hell to Hormone Well* and *From Belly Fat to Belly Flat*. These both provide excellent information on natural approaches to hormone health.

There are many other physician pioneers and medical experts who have helped lay a foundation of learning and knowledge regarding bioidentical hormone therapy. We have the following books in our personal library. Each author offers the reader the benefit of additional information and another perspective. Please note that these resources are not prioritized by perceived merit but are listed in alphabetical order according to author.

Lee, John R. *Natural Progesterone, The Multiple Role of a Remarkable Hormone.* Sebastopol, CA: BLL Publishing, 1993.

Lee, John R., with Jesse Hanley and Virginia Hopkins. *What Your Doctor May NOT Tell You About Perimenopause.* New York: Warner Books, 1999.

Lee, John R., with Virginia Hopkins. *What Your Doctor May NOT Tell You About Menopause.* New York: Warner Books, 1996.

Lee, John R., with David Zava and Virginia Hopkins. *What Your Doctor May NOT Tell You About Breast Cancer.* New York: Warner Books, 2002.

Northrup, Christiane. *Women's Bodies, Women's Wisdom: Creating Physical and Emotional Health and Healing.* New York: Bantam Books, 1994.

Northrup, Christiane. *The Wisdom of Menopause: Creating Physical and Emotional Health and Healing During the Change.* New York: Bantam Books, 2001.

Schwartz, Erika. *The Hormone Solution.* New York: Warner Books, 2002.

Seaman, Barbara. *The Greatest Experiment Ever Performed on Women: Exploding the Estrogen Myth.* New York: Hyperion Books, 2003.

Shulman, Neil, and Kim S. Edmunds. *Healthy Transitions: A Woman's Guide to Perimenopause, Menopause & Beyond.* New York: Prometheus Books, 2004.

Somers, Suzanne. *The Sexy Years, Discover the Hormone Connection: The*

Secret to Fabulous Sex, Great Health, and Vitality for Women and Men. New York: Crown Publishers, 2004.

Taylor, Eldred, and Ava Bell-Taylor. *Are Your Hormones Making You Sick?* Orlando, FL: Physicians Natural Medicine, 2000.

Whitaker, Julian. *Dr. Whitaker's Guide to Natural Hormone Replacement.* Potomac, MD: Phillips Publishing, 1999.

Wilson, James L. *Adrenal Fatigue.* Petaluma, CA: Smart Publications, 2003.

Wright, Jonathan V., and John Morgenthaler. *Natural Hormone Replacement for Women Over 45.* Petaluma, CA: Smart Publications, 1997.

Newsletters

E-mail newsletters can be a great source of new information regarding hormone health. They can also serve as excellent reminders of good information you might have read once but have forgotten. There are several excellent newsletters available today. I recommend that you check out/sign up for:

- Our free monthly newsletter. Go to www.hormonewell.com to register.
- Virginia Hopkin's Healthwatch: healthwatch@virginiahopkins healthwatch.com.
- Women in Balance: www.womeninbalance.org.

Best Resource: Yourself

In closing, I want to take a minute to remind each reader that no one can tell you what is right for you, your body, or your health. I encourage you to read, ask questions, and do your homework. While it is our privilege to be your resource, only you can be your own final authority when it comes to your health and well-being.

NOTES

Chapter 1

1. William A Marshall and JM Tanner "Puberty," in F. Falkner and JM Tanner, eds. *Human Growth: A Comprehensive Treatise,* 2nd ed. New York: Plenum Press (1986), 171–209.
2. DB Adams, AR Gold, and AD Burt. Rise in female initiated sexual activity at ovulation and its suppression by oral contraceptives. *New England Journal of Medicine* 299 (1978): 1145–1150.
3. Homa Keshavarz, Susan D Hillis, Burney A Kieke, and Polly A Marchbanks. Centers for Disease Control, Surveillance Summaries: Hysterectomy Surveillance, United States 1994–1999. 51(SS05) (July 12, 2002): 1–8.
4. Endogenous Hormones and Breast Cancer Collaborative Group. Free estradiol and breast cancer risk in postmenopausal women. *Cancer Epidemiology Biomarkers & Prevention* 12 (2003): 1457–1461.
5. RB Wallace, BM Sherman, JA Bean, JP Leeper, and AE Treloar. Menstrual cycle patterns and breast cancer risk factors. *Medline* 11, part 2 (1978): 4021–4024.

6. Cheryl L Rock, Shirley W Flatt, Gail A Laughlin, Ellen B Gold, Cynthia A Thomson, Loki Natarajan, Lovell A Jones, Bette J Caan, Marcia L Stefanick, Richard A Hajek, Wael K Al-Delaimy, Frank Z Stanczyk, and John P Pierce. Reproductive steroid hormones and recurrence-free survival in women with a history of breast cancer. *Cancer Epidemiology, Biomarkers & Prevention* 17 (2008): 614–620.

7. P Multi, HL Bradlow, A Micheli, V Krogh, JL Freudenheim, HJ Schunemann, M Stanulla, J Yang, DW Sepkovic, M Trevisan, and F. Berrino. Estrogen metabolism and risk of breast cancer: a prospective study of the 2:16alpha-hydroxyestrone ration in premenopausal and postmenopausal women. *Epidemiology* 11(6) (2000): 635–640.

8. JA Cauley, JM Zmuda, ME Danielson, BM Ljung, DC Bauer, SR Cummings, and LH Kuller. Estrogen metabolites and the risk of breast cancer in older women. *Epidemiology* 14(6) (2003): 740–744.

9. S Rako. Testosterone deficiency: a key factor in the increased cardiovascular risk to women following hysterectomy or with natural aging? *Journal of Women's Health* 7(7) (1998): 825–829.

10. Erik Debing, Els Peeters, William Duquet, Kris Poppe, Brigitte Velkeniers, and Pierre Van den Brande. Endogenous sex hormone levels in postmenopausal women undergoing carotid artery endarterectomy. *European Journal of Endocrinology* 156(6) (2007): 687–693.

Chapter 2

1. Available at www.census.gov/ipc/www/usinterimproj/natprojtab02a.pdf.

2. Melissa Conrad Stoppler. Puberty. MedicineNet.com (2009).

3. Kay-Tee Khaw, Mitch Dowsett, Elizabeth Folkerd, Sheila Bingham, Nicholas Wareham, Robert Luben, Ailsa Welch, and Nicholas Day. Endogenous testosterone and mortality due to all causes, cardiovascular disease and cancer in men. *Circulation* 116 (2007): 2694–2701.

4. T Hugh Jones. Testosterone—clinical associations with the metabolic syndrome and type 2 diabetes mellitus. *European Endocrine Disease* 1 (2007): 799–806.

5. Ibid.

6. EL Rhoden and A Morgentaler. Risks of testosterone-replacement

therapy and recommendations for monitoring. *New England Journal of Medicine* 350 (2004): 482–492.

7. William R Carpenter, Whitney R Robinson, and Paul A Godley. Getting over testosterone: postulating a fresh start for etiologic studies of prostate cancer. *Journal of the National Cancer Institute* 100(3) (2008): 158–159.

8. Abraham Morgentaler. *Testosterone for Life.* New York: McGraw-Hill (2009), 123.

9. Eric Orwoll, Lori C Lambert, Lynn M Marshall, Janet Blank, Elizabeth Barrett-Connor, Jane Cauley, Kris Ensrud, and Steven R Cummings, for the Osteoporotic Fractures in Men Study Group. Endogenous testosterone levels, physical performance, and fall risk in older men. *Archives of Internal Medicine* 166 (2006): 2124–2131.

10. Elizabeth M Haney, Benjamin KS Chan, Susan J Diem, Kristine E Ensrud, Jane A Cauley, Elizabeth Barrett-Connor, Eric Orwoll, and M Michael Bliziotes, for the Osteoporotic Fractures in Men Study Group. Association of low bone mineral density with selective serotonin reuptake inhibitor use by older men. *Archives of Internal Medicine* 167 (2007): 1246–1251.

11. OP Almeida, BB Yeap, GJ Hankey, K Jamrozik, and L Flicker. Low free testosterone concentration as a potentially treatable cause of depressive symptoms in older men. *Archives of General Psychiatry* 65(3) (2008): 283–289.

12. Sandeep Saluja. DHEA: an enigmatic medicine. *Internet Journal of Endocrinology* 2(2) (2006). www.ispub.com/journal/theinternetjournalof endocrinology/volume2number216/article.

Chapter 3

1. RS Vasan, MJ Pencina, M Cobian, MS Freiberg, and RB D'Agostino. Estimated risks for developing obesity in the Framingham Heart Study. *Annals of Internal Medicine* 143, (2005): 473–480.

2. Megan A McCrory, Vivian MM Suen, and Susan B Roberts. Biobehavioral influences on energy intake and adult weight gain. *Journal of Nutrition* 132 (2002): 3830S–3834S.

3. Colette Bouchez. Better sex: what's weight got to do with it? *Journal of Sex and Marital Therapy* 26 (2000): 191–208.

4. Rhea Seymour. Libido killers. *Flare* (August 2007).

5. Lisa Martinez. *Women's Sexual Health Journal* 18 (October 2008): 1–11.

6. Consumer Reports poll: economy isn't hurting Americans' sex lives. *Consumer Reports Health* (2007). www.consumerreports.org/health/medical_conditions_treatments/sexpoll/overview/sex_poll_ov.htm.

7. We're not in the mood. www.nomarriage.com/articlesexless.html, June 30, 2008.

8. Robert T Michael, John H Gagnon, Edward O Laumann, and Gina Kolata. *Sex in America: A Definitive Survey.* Boston: Little Brown (1994).

9. Lynne Lamberg. Most Americans seldom get a good night's sleep. *Psychiatric News* 40(10) (2005): 35.

10. E Carlsen, A Giwwercman, N Keiding, and N Skakkebaek. Evidence for decreasing quality of semen during past 50 years. *British Medical Journal* 305 (1992): 609–613.

11. Cynthia A Graham, John Bancroft, Helen A Doll, Theresa Greco, and Amanda Tanner. Does oral contraceptive–induced reduction in free testosterone adversely affect the sexuality or mood of women? *Psychoneuroendocrinology* 32(3) (2007): 246–255.

12. Laura Berman. *Real Sex for Real Women.* Singapore: DK Adult (2008), 20.

Chapter 4

1. Cathy Seltzer. Fourth annual top 50 *Pharma. Exec.* special report. *Pharmaceutical Executive* (May 2003): 45.

2. Shirley S. Wang and Sarah Rubenstein. Wyeth is pressed on drug reviews. *Wall Street Journal* (December 13–14, 2008).

3. Barbara Seaman. *The Greatest Experiment Ever Performed on Women.* New York: Hyperion (2003), 28.

4. Robert Koenig. Reopening the darkest chapter in German science. *Science* (June 3, 2000).

5. Susan Benedict and Jane M Georges. Nurses and the sterilization experiment of Auschwitz: a postmodernist perspective. *Nursing Inquiry* 13(4) (2006): 277–288.

6. Avrum Z Bluming. A decline in breast-cancer incidence. *New England Journal of Medicine* 357(5) (2007): 509–513.

7. Gerardo Heiss, Robert Wallace, Garnet L Anderson, Aaron Aragaki, Shirley AA Beresford, Robert Brzyski, Rowan T Chlebowski, Margery

Gass, Andrea LaCroix, JoAnn E Manson, Ross L Prentice, Jacques Rossouw, and Marcia L Stefanick; for the WHI investigators. Health risks and benefits 3 years after stopping randomized treatment with estrogen and progestin. *Journal of the American Medical Association* 299(9) (2008): 989–1096.

8. Federation of European Cancer Societies. The pill may increase risk of breast cancer, according to large study of younger women. *Science Daily* (2002).

9. For information on the Billings ovulation method, visit www.boma _usa.org.

Chapter 5

1. R Raz and WE Stamm. A controlled trial of intravaginal estriol in postmenopausal women with recurrent urinary tract infections. *New England Journal of Medicine* 329(111) (1993): 753–756.

2. Erik Debing, Els Peeters, William Duquet, Kris Poppe, Brigitte Velkeniers, and Pierre Van den Baarde. Endogenous sex hormones levels in postmenopausal women undergoing carotid artery endosterectomy. *European Journal of Endocrinology* 156(6): 687–693.

3. Dimitrakakis C, Zhou J, Wang J, et al. A physiologic role for testosterone in limiting estrogenic stimulation of the breast. *Menopause.* 10(4) (2003): 292–298.

4. Elmer M Cranton and William Fryer. Testosterone replacement: the male andropause. In *Resetting the Clock*, Lanham, MD: Roman Littlefield, (1997).

5. Abraham Morgentaler. *Testosterone for Life.* New York: McGraw-Hill (2009), 135.

Chapter 6

1. Steven F Hotze. A revolution in wellness. www.hotzehwc.com.

2. The Casey Group. Is bioidentical hormone therapy for you? www.body logicmd.com.

3. Mayo Clinic Staff. Human growth hormone (HGH): does it slow aging? www.mayoclinic.com (2009).

4. Jennifer Goodrum. Estriol: women's choice vs. a manufacturer's greed. *International Journal of Pharmaceutical Compounding* 12(4) (2008): 286–294.
5. Joann V Pinkerton. Bioidentical hormones: what you (and your patient) need to know. *OBG Management* 21(01) (2009): 42–52.

Chapter 7

1. The new hormone replacement therapy *Life Extension Magazine* (December 2002). www.lef.org/magazine/may2002/dec2002_report _hormone_02.html.
2. Marcelle Pick. Phytotherapy—the key to hormonal balance? www .womentowomen.com (2008/2009).
3. F Branca and S Lorenzetti. Health effects of phytoestrogens. *Forum Nutrition* 57 (2005): 100–111.
4. CI Madding, M Jacob, VP Ramsay, and RZ Sokol. Serum and semen zinc levels in normozoospermic and oligozoospermic men. *Annals of Nutrition and Metabolism* 30(4) (1986): 213–218.
5. University of Maryland Medical Center. Omega-3 fatty acids. www .umm.edu/altmed/articles/omega-3-00031b.htm.
6. J Narbonne et al. Protein metabolism in vitamin A deficient rats. II. Protein synthesis in striated muscle. *Annales de la nutrition et de l'alimentation* 32(1) (1978): 59–75.
7. T Fususho et al. Tissue-specific distribution and metabolism of vitamin A are affected by dietary protein levels in rats. *International Journal for Vitamin and Nutrition Research* 68(5) (1998): 287–292.

Chapter 8

1. David M Eisenberg, Ronald C Kessler, Cindy Foster, Frances E Norlock, David R Calkins, and Thomas L Delbanco. Unconventional medicine in the United States—prevalence, costs and patterns of use. *New England Journal of Medicine* 328(4) (1993): 246–252.
2. David M Eisenberg. Complementary and alternative medicine in the United States: overview and patterns of use. *Journal of Alternative and Complementary Medicine* 7(1) (2001): S19–S21.

3. Licorice. *University of Maryland Medical Center* (2007).
   Y Abe, T Ueda, T Kato, et al. Female hormone replacement therapy. *Nippon Rinsho* 52(7) (1994): 1817–1822.
4. F Sheu, H Lai, and G-C Yen. Suppression effect of soy isoflavones on nitric oxide production. *Journal of Agricultural and Food Chemistry* 49(4) (2001): 1767–1772.
5. A Huntley and E Ernst. A systematic review of the safety of black cohosh. *Journal of the North American Menopause Society* 10(1) (2003): 58–64.
6. National Center for Complimentary Medicine. Black cohosh at a glance (November 2008), www.nccam.nih.gov/health/blackcohosh/ataglance.htm.

Chapter 9

1. GF Gonzales, A Cordova, K Vega, et al. Effect of *Lepidium meyenii* (maca), a root with aphrodisiac and fertility-enhancing properties, on serum reproductive hormone levels in adult healthy men. *Journal of Endocrinology* 176(1) (2003): 163–168.
2. Dale Kiefer. Improving vitality, sexual function, and prostate health in aging men. *Life Extension* 14(12) (2008): 27–28.
3. CM Dording, L. Fisher, G. Papakostas, et al. A double-blind randomized, pilot dose-finding study of maca root *(L. meyenii)* for the management of SSRI-induced sexual dysfunction. *Central Nervous System Neuroscience Therapy* 14(3) (2008): 182–191.
4. CH Oliveira, ME Moraes, MO Moraes, et al. Clinical toxicology study of an herbal medicinal extract of *Paullinia cupana, Trichilia catigua, Ptychopetalum olacoides* and *Zingiber officinale* (catuama) in healthy volunteers. *Phytotherapy Research* 19(1) (2005): 54–57.
5. J Waynberg. Yohimbine vs. muira puama in the treatment of sexual dysfunction. *American Journal of Natural Medicine* 1 (1994): 8–9.
6. IR Siqueira, C Fochesatto, AL da Silva, et al. Ptychopetalum olacoides, a traditional Amazonian "nerve tonic," possesses anticholinesterase activity. *Pharmacology Biochemistry and Behaviour* 75(3) (2003): 645–650.
7. Dale Kiefer. Nettle and ginger. *Life Extension* 14(12) (2008): 30.
8. E Giovannucci, et al. Intake of carotenoids and retinal in relation to risk of prostate cancer. *Journal of the National Cancer Institute* 87(23) (1995): 1766–1776.

9. DL Rowland and W Tai. A review of plant-derived and herbal approaches to the treatment of sexual dysfunction. *Journal of Sex and Marital Therapy* 29 (2003): 185–205.

10. TY Ito, AS Trant, and ML Polan. A double-blind placebo-controlled study of ArginMax, a nutritional supplement for enhancement of female sexual function. *Journal of Sex and Marriage Therapy* 27(5) (2001): 541–549.

11. CM Meston and M Worcel. The effects of yohimbine plus L-arginine glutamate on sexual arousal in postmenopausal women with sexual arousal disorder. *Archives of Sexual Behavior* 31(4) (2002): 323–332.

12. A Cohen. Treatment of antidepressant-induced sexual dysfunction with ginkgo biloba extract. *New Research Report from the Proceedings of the American Psychiatric Association Annual Meeting* 716 (1996).

13. J Waynberg. Contributions to the clinical validation of the traditional use of ptychopetalum guyanna. Presented at the First International Congress of Ethnopharmacology, Strasbourg, France, June 5–9, 1990.

14. AL da Silva, ALS Piato, S Bardini, et al. Memory retrieval improvement by *Ptychopetalum Olacoides* in young and aging mice. *Journal of Ethnopharmacology* 95(2–3) (2004): 199–203.

Chapter 10

1. JD MacDougall, CE Webber, J Martin, S Ormerod, A Chesley, EV Younglai, CL Gordon, and CJ Blimkie. Relationship among running mileage, bone density, and serum testosterone in male runners. *Journal of Applied Physiology* 733 (1992): 1165–1170.

2. Michael D Roberts, Mike Iosia, Chad M Kerksick, Lem W Taylor, Bill Campbell, Colin D Wilborn, Travis Harvey, Matthew Cooke, Chris Rasmussen, Mike Greenwood, Ronald Wilson, Jean Jitomir, Darryn Willoughby, and Richard B Kreider. Effects of arachidonic acid supplementation on training adaptation in resistance-trained males. *Journal of the International Society of Sports Nutrition* 4 (2007): 21.

3. National Orgasm Day 31 July 2008—The 2008 Orgasm Survey. *Scientific Blogging* (2008).

4. Amy Painter. Exercises to improve your sex life. *Discovery Health* (2009).

5. Lisa Dawn Hamilton, Alessandra H Rellini, and Cindy M Meston. Cortisol, sexual arousal, and affect in response to sexual stimuli. *J Sex Med* 5 (2008): 2111–2118.

6. Constance G Bacon, Murray A Mittleman, Ichiro Kawachi, Edward Giovannucci, Dale B Glasser, and Eric B Rimm. Sexual function in men older than 50 years of age: results from the Health Professionals Follow-up Study. *Annals of Internal Medicine* 139(3) (2003): 161–168.

7. Tina M Penhollow and Michael Young. Sexual desirability and sexual performance: does exercise and fitness really matter? *Electronic Journal of Human Sexuality* 7 (2004).

8. Katherine Esposito, Francesco Giugliano, Carmen Di Palo, Giovanni Giugliano, Raffaele Marfella, Francesco D'Andrea, Massimo D'Armiento, and Dario Giugliano. Effect of lifestyle changes on erectile dysfunction in obese men. A randomized controlled trial. *Journal of the American Medical Association* 291(24) (2004): 2978–2984.

9. Tina M Penhollow and Michael Young. Sexual desirability and sexual performance: does exercise and fitness really matter? *Electronic Journal of Human Sexuality* 7 (2004).

Chapter 11

1. Sexercise. www.today.ninemsn.com.

2. R Doll. One for the heart. *British Medical Journal* 315 (1997): 1664–1668.

3. Kathleen Doheny. Top 10 reasons to have sex tonight. *CBS News* (March 24, 2008).

4. Shelley E Taylor, Laura Cousino Kelin, Brian P Lewis, Tara L Gruenewald, Regan AR Gurung, and John A Updegraff. Biobehavioral responses to stress in females: tend-and-befriend, not fight-or-flight. *Psychological Review* 107(3) (2000): 411–429.

5. Michael F Leitzmann, Elizabeth A Platz, Meir J Stampfer, Walter C Willett, and Edward Giovannucci. Ejaculation frequency and subsequent risk of prostate cancer. *Journal of the American Medical Association* 291(13) (2004): 1578–1586.

6. Douglas Fox. Masturbating may protect against prostate cancer, July 16, 2003.

7. Christian Unkelbach, Adam J Guastella, and Joseph P Forgas. Oxytocin selectively facilitates recognition of positive sex and relationship words. *Psychology Science Journal* 19(11) (2008): 1092–1094.

8. Hormone oxytocin makes you trust strangers more with your money.

Medical News Today (June 3, 2005), www.medicalnewstoday.com/articles/25559.php.

9. AT Bodley-Tickell, B Olowokure, S Bhaduri, DJ White, D Ward, JDC Ross, G Smith, HV Duggal, and P Goold, on behalf of the West Midlands STI Surveillance Project. Epidemiology, trends in sexually transmitted infections (other than HIV) in older people: analysis of data from an enhanced surveillance system. *Sexually Transmitted Infections* 84 (2008): 312–317.

REFERENCES

Chapter 1

L Baker, KK Meldrum, M Wang, R Sankula, R Vanam, A Raiesdana, B Tsai, K Hile, JW Brown, and DR Meldrum. The role of estrogen in cardiovascular disease. *Journal of Surgical Research* 115 (2003): 325–344.

TL Bush and E Barrett-Connor. Noncontraceptive estrogen use and cardiovascular disease. *Epidemiologic Reviews* 7 (1985): 89–104.

JA Cauley, JP Gutai, NW Glynn, M Paternostro-Bayles, E Cottington, and LH Kuller. Serum estrone concentrations and coronary artery disease in postmenopausal women. *Arteriosclerosis, Thrombosis and Vascular Biology* 14 (1994): 14–18.

IF Godsland, V Wynn, D Crook, and NE Miller. Sex, plasma lipoproteins, and atherosclerosis: prevailing assumptions and outstanding questions. *American Heart Journal* 114 (1987): 1467–1503.

KL Irwin, HB Peterson, JM Hughes, and SW Gill. Hysterectomy among women of reproductive age, United States updated for 1981–1982. In CDC surveillance summaries. *Morbidity and Mortality Weekly Report* 35 (ISS) (1986): 1SS–6SS.

LA Lepine, SD Hillis, PA Marchbank, et al. Hysterectomy surveillance—United States, 1980–1993. In CDC surveillance summaries. *Morbidity and Mortality Weekly Report* 46 (SS-4) (1997): 1–16.

CJ Malkin, PJ Pugh, RD Jones, TH Jones, and KS Channer. Testosterone as a protective factor against atherosclerosis—immunomodulation and influence upon plaque development and stability. *Journal of Endocrinology* 178 (2003): 373–380.

Margaret RH Nusbaum, Armit R Singh, and Amanda A Pyles. Sexual healthcare needs of women aged 65 and older. *Journal of the American Geriatrics Society* 52 (2004): 117–122.

GB Phillips, BH Pinkernell, and TY Jing. Relationship between serum sex hormones and coronary artery disease in postmenopausal women. *Arthrosclerosis, Thrombosis and Vascular Biology* 17 (1997): 695–701.

Erika Schwartz. *The Hormone Solution.* Grand Central Publishing. New York: (2002).

K Wallen. Periovulatory changes in female sexual behavior and patterns of ovarian steroid secretion in group-living rhesus monkeys. *Hormones and Behavior* 18(4) (1984): 431–450.

FC Wu and A von Eckardstein. Androgens and coronary artery disease. *Endocrine Reviews* 24 (2003): 183–217.

Chapter 2

CA Allan and RI McLachan. Age-related changes in testosterone and the role of replacement therapy in older men. *Clinical Endocrinology* 60 (2004): 653–670.

CA Allan, BJ Strauss, and RI McLachlan. Body composition, metabolic syndrome and testosterone in aging men. *International Journal of Impotence Research* 19(5) (2007): 448–457.

AB Araujo, AB O'Donnell, DJ Brambilla, WB Simpson, C Longcope, AM Matsumoto, et al. Prevalence and incidence of androgen deficiency in middle-age and older men: estimates from the MMAS. *Journal of Clinical Endocrinology and Metabolism* 89(12) (2004): 5920–5926.

A Aversa, AM Isidors, G Spera, A Lenzi, and A Fabbri. Androgens improve vasodilation and response to sildenafil in patients with erectile dysfunction. *Clinical Endocrinology* 58(5) (2003): 632–638.

CJ Bagatell and WJ Bremner. Androgen and progestagen effects on plasma lipids. *Progress in Cardiovascular Diseases* 38(3) (1995): 255–271.

EE Baulieu, G Thomas, S Legrain, N Lahlou, M Roger, B Debuire, V Faucounau, L Girard, MP Hervy, F Latour, MC Leaud, A Mokrane, H Pitti-

Ferrandi, C Trivalle, O de Lacharriere, S Nouveau, B Rakoto-Arison, JC Souberbielle, J Raison, Y Le Bouc, A Raynaud, X Girerd, and F Forette. Dehydroepiandrosterone (DHEA), DHEA sulfate, and aging: contribution of the DHEA Age Study to a sociobiomedical issue. *Proceedings of the National Academy of Sciences of the United States of America* 97(8) (2000): 4279–4284.

Cancer risk: analysis of individual patient data from 12 prospective studies. *Annals of Internal Medicine* 149(7) (2008): 461–471.

Malcom Carruthers. *The Testosterone Revolution.* London: Thorsons (2001).

MM Cherrier, BD Anawalt, KL Herbst, et al. Cognitive effects of short-term manipulation of serum sex steroids in healthy young men. *Journal of Clinical Endocrinology and Metabolism* 87(7) (2002): 3090–3096.

MM Cherrier, S Plymate, S Mohan, et al., Relationship between testosterone supplementation and insulin-like growth factor-I levels and cognition in healthy older men. *Psychoneuroendocrinology* 29(1) (2004): 65–82.

FW Danby. Endogenous sex hormones and prostate cancer: a collaborative analysis of 18 prospective studies. *Journal of the National Cancer Institute* 100(19) (2008): 1412–1413.

S Dhindsa, S Prabhakar, M Sethi, A Bandyopadhyay, A Chaudhuri, and P Dandona. Frequent occurrence of hypogonodatropic hypogonadism in type 2 diabetes. *Journal of Clinical Endocrinology and Metabolism* 89(11) (2004): 5462–5468.

European Journal of Endocrinology. Investigation, treatment and monitoring of late-onset hypogonadism in males: ISA, ISSAM, EAU, EAA and ASA recommendations. *Oxford Journals* 159(5) (2008): 507–514.

ER Freeman, DA Bloom, and EJ McGuire. A brief history of testosterone. *Journal of Urology* 165(2) (2001): 371–373.

A Gray, HA Feldman, JB McKinlay, and C Longscope. Age, disease and changing sex hormone levels in middle-aged men: results of the Massachusetts Male Aging Study. *Journal of Clinical Endocrinology and Metabolism* 73 (1991): 1016–1025.

CG Heller and G Myers. The male climacteric, its symptomatology, diagnosis and treatment. *Journal of the American Medical Association* 126(8) (1944): 472–477.

AW Hsing, LW Chu, and FZ Stanczyk. Androgen and prostate cancer: is the hypothesis dead? *Cancer Epidemiology Biomarkers and Prevention* 17(10) (2008): 2525–2530.

IOM. *Testosterone and Aging: Clinical Research Directions.* Washington, DC: Institute of Medicine (2003).

RR Kalyani and AS Dobs. Androgen deficiency, diabetes, and the metabolic syndrome in older men. *Current Opinion in Endocrinology, Diabetes and Obesity* 14(3) (2007): 226–234.

AM Kenny, KM Prestwood, CA Gruman, KM Marcello, and LG Raisz. Effects of transdermal testosterone on bone and muscle in older men with low bioavailable testosterone levels. *Journals of Gerontology Series A: Biological Sciences and Medical Sciences* 56(5) (2001): M266–M272.

KT Khaw, M. Dowsett, E. Folkerd, et al. Endogenous testosterone and mortality due to all causes, cardiovascular disease, and cancer in men: European prospective investigation into cancer in Norfolk (EPIC-Norfolk) Prospective Population Study. *Circulation* 116(23) (2007): 2694–2701.

John R. Lee. *Male Menopause.* Windsor, CA: Hormones, Etc. (2003).

AM Matsumoto. Andropause: clinical implications of the decline in serum testosterone levels with aging in men. *Journals of Gerontology Series A: Biological Sciences and Medical Sciences* 57(2) (2002): M76–M99.

MM Miner and AD Seftel. Testosterone and ageing: what have we learned since the Institute of Medicine report and what lies ahead? *International Journal of Clinical Practice* 61(4) (2007): 622–632.

A Morgentaler. Male impotence. *Lancet* 354 (1999): 1713–1718.

A Morgentaler, CO Bruning III, and WC DeWolf. Incidence of occult prostate cancer among men with low total or free serum testosterone. *Journal of the American Medical Association* 276 (1996): 1904–1906.

A Morgentaler and D Crews. Role of the anterior hypothalamus-preoptic area in the regulation of reproductive behavior in the lizard, *Anolis carolinensis:* implantation studies. *Hormones and Behavior* 11 (2006): 61.

A Morgentaler and EL Rhoden. Prevalence of prostate cancer among hypogonadal men with prostate-specific antigen of 4.0 ng/mL or less. *Urology* 68 (2006): 1263–1267.

JE Morley. Andropause, testosterone therapy, and quality of life in aging men. *Cleveland Clinic Journal of Medicine* 67(12) (2000): 880–882.

JE Morley and HM Perry. Andropause: an old concept in new clothing. *Clinics in Geriatric Medicine* 19(3) (2003): 507–528.

MI Naharci, M Pinar, E Bolu, and A Olgun. Effect of testosterone on insulin sensitivity in men with idiopathic hypogonadotropic hypogonadism. *Endocrine Practice* 13(6) (2007): 629–635.

WJ Reiter, G Schatzl, I Mark, A Zeiner, A Pycha, and M Marberger. Dehydroepiandrosterone in the treatment of erectile dysfunction in patients with different organic etiologies. *Urology Research* 29(4) (2001): 278–281.

EL Rhoden and A Morgentaler. Risks of testosterone-replacement therapy and recommendations for monitoring. *New England Journal of Medicine* 350 (2004): 482–492.

AW Roddam, NE Allen, P Appleby, TJ Key, L Ferrucci, HB Carter, EJ Metter, C Chen, NS Weiss, A Fitzpatrick, et al. Insulin-like growth factors, their binding proteins, and prostate. *Annals of Internal Medicine,* 149(7) (2008): 461–471.

Marc R Rose, ML Black, ML Lowenstein, and V Hopkins. *A Woman's Guide to Male Menopause.* Connecticut: Keats Publishing (2001).

SN Seidman. Testosterone deficiency and mood in aging men: pathogenic and therapeutic interactions. *World Journal of Biological Psychiatry* 4(1) (2003): 14–20.

Eugene Shippen. *The Testosterone Syndrome.* New York: M. Evans & Co. (1998).

RF Spark. Testosterone, diabetes mellitus, and the metabolic syndrome. *Current Urology Reports* 8(6) (2007): 467–471.

SN Stas, AG Anastasiadis, H Fisch, MC Benson, and R Shabsigh. Urologic aspects of andropause. *Urology* 61(2) (2003): 261–266.

RS Tan. Memory loss as a reported symptom of andropause. *Archives of Andrology* 47 (2001): 185–189.

RS Tan. Andropause: introducing the concept of "relative hypogonadism" in aging males. *International Journal of Impotence Research* 14(4) (2002): 319.

RS Tan and JW Culberson. An integrative review on current evidence of testosterone replacement therapy for the andropause. *Maturitas* 45(1) (2003): 15–27.

RS Tan and PS Philip. Perceptions of and risk factors for andropause. *Archives of Andrology* 43(2) (1999): 97–103.

RS Tan and SJ Pu. The andropause and memory loss: is there a link between androgen decline and dementia in the aging male? *Asian Journal Andrology* 3 (2001): 169–174.

RS Tan and SJ Pu. Is it andropause? Recognizing androgen deficiency in aging men. *Postgraduate Medicine* 115(1) (2004):62–66.

RS Tan, SJ Pu, and JW Culberson. Role of androgens in mild cognitive (thinking) impairment and possible interventions during andropause. *Medical Hypotheses* 62(1) (2004): 14–18.

Testosterone and Aging: Clinical Research Directions. Washington, DC: Institute of Medicine (2003).

AA Werner. The male climacteric: report of 273 cases. *Journal of the American Medical Association* 132 (1946): 188–194.

E Wespes and CC Schulmann. Male andropause: myth, reality and treatment. *International Journal of Impotence Research* 14 (2002): S93–S98.

Chapter 3

Steven C Abell and Maryse H Richards. The relationship between body shape satisfaction and self-esteem: an investigation of gender and class differences. *Journal of Youth and Adolescence* 25(5) (1996): 691.

N Allon. "The Stigma of Overweight in Everyday Life," in BB Wolman, ed. *Psychological Aspect's of Obesity: A Handbook.* New York: Van Norstrand Reighold (1982), 130–174.

John Bancroft. Biological factors in human sexuality. *Journal of Sex Research* 39(1) (2002): 114–126.

John Bancroft. *Human Sexuality and Its Problems,* 3rd ed. Edinburgh, Scotland: Churchill Livingston Elsevier (2009).

M Binks. Sexual problems common among obese people. *WebMD* (2004).

Sara K Bridges, Suzanne H Lease, and Carol R Ellison. Predicting sexual satisfaction in women: implications for counselor education and training. *Journal of Counseling and Development* 82(2) (2004): 158.

H Cookson. Not in the mood? Young women don't want to talk about it, but a lack of sexual desire is common. Here are some surprising causes and solutions from sexperts. Woodland Hills, CA: *Weider Publications* (2004).

M Crawford and D Poop. Sexual double standards: a review and methodological critique of two decades of research. *Journal of Sex Research* 40(1) (2003): 13.

Michelle Dionne, Carolin Davis, John Fox, and Maria Gurevich. Feminist ideology as a predictor of body dissatisfaction in women. *Sex Roles: A Journal of Research* 33(3–4) (1995): 277.

Forssman-Falck, W Kilmartin Kliewer, B Myers, and M Polce-Lynch. Gender and age patterns in emotional expression, body image and self-esteem: a qualitative analysis. *Sex Roles: A Journal of Research* 38(1025) (1988): 11–12.

LR Fraser, et al. Effects of estradiol 17B and environmental estrogens on mammalian sperm function. Presented at the annual conference of the European Society of Human Reproduction and Embryology, Vienna (2002).

Ilona Gossmann, Mireille Mathieu, Danielle Julien, and Elise Chartrand. Determinants of sex initiation frequencies and sexual satisfaction in long-term couples' relationships. *Canadian Journal of Human Sexuality* 12(169) (2003): 3–4.

J Loftus and JS Long. Distress about sex: a national survey of women in heterosexual relationships. *Archives of Sexual Behavior* 32(3) (2003): 193.

JC Lovejoy. The influence of sex hormones on obesity across the female life span. *Women's Health* 7(10) (1998): 1247–1256.

SL Woodward. Factors in sexual satisfaction of obese women in relationships. *Electronic Journal of Human Sexuality* 5 (2002).

Chapter 4

American College of Obstetricians and Gynecologists. Risk of breast cancer with estrogen-progestin replacement therapy. *International Journal of Gynecology and Obstetrics* 76 (2002): 333–335.

Susan Benedict and Jane M Georges. Nurses and the sterilization experiments of Auschwitz: a postmodernist perspective. *Nursing Inquiry* 13(4) (2006): 277–288.

M Bibbo, WM Haenszel, GL Wied, M Hubby, and AL Herbst. A twenty-five year follow-up study of women exposed to diethylstilbestrol during pregnancy. *New England Journal of Medicine* 298(14) (1978): 763–767.

MM Braun, A Ahlbom, B Floderus, LA Brinton, and RN Hoover. Effect of twinship in incidence of cancer of the testis, breasts, and other sites [Sweden]. *Cancer Causes Control* 6 (1995): 519–524.

DD Brian, BC Tilley, DR Labarthe, WM O'Fallon, KL Noller, and LT Kurland. Breast cancer in DES-exposed mothers—absence of association. *Mayo Clinic Proceedings* 55 (1980): 89–93.

BM Caldwell and RI Watson. An evaluation of psychologic effects of sex hormone administration in aged women: results of therapy after six months. *Journal of Gerontology* (1952): 228.

Rowan T Chlebowski, Susan L Hendrix, Robert D Langer, Marcia L Stefanick, Margery Gass, Dorothy Lane, Rebecca J Rodabough, Mary Ann Gilligan, Michele G. Cyr, Cynthia A Thomson, Janardan Khandekar,

Helen Petrovitch, and Anne McTiernan, for the WHI Investigators. Influence of estrogen plus progestin on breast cancer and mammography in healthy postmenopausal women. *Journal of the American Medical Association* 289 (24) (2003):

Collaborative Group on Hormonal Factors in Breast Cancer. Breast cancer and hormone replacement therapy: collaborative reanalysis of data from 51 epidemiological studies of 52,705 women with breast cancer and 108,411 women without breast cancer. *Lancet* 350 (1997): 1047–1059.

Beral V Colwell. Randomized trial of high doses of stilbestrol and ethisterone in pregnancy: long-term follow-up of mothers. *British Medical Journal* 281 (1980): 1098–1101.

CL Dillis and JS Schreiman. Change in mammographic breast density associated with the use of Depo-Provera. *Breast Journal* 9(4) (2003): 312–315.

Peter H Gann and Monica Morrow. Combined hormone therapy and breast cancer: a single-edged sword. *Journal of the American Medical Association* 289(24) (2003): 3304–3306.

N Gavin, J Thorp, and R Oshfeldt. Determinants of hormone replacement therapy duration among postmenopausal women with intact uteri. *Menopause* 8 (2001): 377–383.

GR Gillson and DT Zava. Perspective on hormone replacement for women: picking up the pieces after the Women's Health Initiative trial. *International Journal of Pharmaceutical Compounding* 7(4) (2003): 250.

GA Greendale, BA Reboussin, A Sie, et al. Effects of estrogen and estrogen-progestin on mammographic parenchymal density. *Annals of Internal Medicine* 130 (1999): 262–269.

Jennifer Haas, Celia P Kaplan, Eric P Gerstenberger, and Karla Kerlikowske. Changes in the use of postmenopausal hormone therapy after the publication of clinical trial results. *Annals of Internal Medicine* 140(3) (2004): 184–188.

OC Hadjimichael, JW Meigs, FW Falcier, WD Thompson, and JT Flannery. Cancer risk among women exposed to exogenous estrogens during pregnancy. *Journal of the National Cancer Institute* 4(4) (1984): 831–834.

Jennifer Hays, et al. Effects of estrogen plus progestin on health-related quality of life. *New England Journal of Medicine* 348 (2003): 1893.

AL Herbst, DC Poskanzer, SJ Robboy, I Friedlander, and RE Scully. A prospective comparison of exposed female offspring with unexposed controls. *New England Journal of Medicine* 292(7) (1975): 334–339.

Lars Holmberg, Ole-Erik Iversen, Carl Mgnus Rudenstam, Mats Hammar, Eero Kumpulainen, Janusz Jaskiewicz, Jacek Jassem, Daria Dobaczewska, Hans E Fjosne, Octavio Peralta, Rodrigo Arriagda, Marit Holmqvist, and Johanna Maenpa, on behalf of the HABITS Study Group. Increased risk of recurrence after hormone replacement therapy in breast cancer survivors. *Journal of the National Cancer Institute* 100 (2008): 475–482.

Hormone replacement therapy and the risk of invasive epithelial ovarian cancer in Swedish women. *Journal of the National Cancer Institute* (2002) 94(7): 497–504.

SA Khan, MA Rogers, KK Khurana, MM Meguid, and PJ Numann. Estrogen receptor expression in benign breast epithelium and breast cancer risk. *Journal of the National Cancer Institute* 84 (1992): 1575–1582.

Robert Koenig. Reopening the darkest chapter in German science. *Science Magazine.* 288(5471) (2000): 1576–1577.

James V Lacey, Jr., et al. Menopausal hormone replacement therapy and risk of ovarian cancer. *Journal of the American Medical Association* 334 (2002): 228.

Christopher I Li, Kathleen E Malone, Peggy L Porter, Noel S Weiss, Mei-Tzu C Tang, Kara L Cushing-Haugen, and Janet R Daling. Relationship between long duration and different regimens of hormone therapy and risk of breast cancer. *Journal of the American Medical Association* 289(24) (2003): 3254–3263.

Manjer J Malina, G Berglund, et al. Increased incidence of small and well-differentiated breast tumors in post-menopausal women following hormone replacement therapy. *Journal of the National Cancer Institute* 92 (2001): 919–922.

Eliza McCarthy. Estrogen uncovered. Have women been the unwitting victims of the medical establishment's experiment with hormones? *Slate* (August 22, 2003), www.slate.com/id/2087317/.

J Meara, M Vessey, and DV Fairweather. A randomized double-blind controlled trial of the value of diethylstilbestrol therapy in pregnancy: 35 years follow-up of mothers and their offspring. *British Journal of Obstetrics and Gynecology* 96(5) (1989): 620–622.

Tobias Millrod, for the Writing Group for the Women's Health Initiative Investigators. Risks and benefits of estrogen plus progestin in healthy post-menopausal women. *Journal of the American Medical Association* 288 (2002): 321–333.

Mosby. *Human Pharmacology,* 3rd ed. St. Louis, MO: Mosby-Year Book (1998).

Benno Muller-Hill. Genetics of susceptibility to tuberculosis: Mengele's experiments in Auschwitz. *Nature Reviews Genetics* 2 (2001): 631–634.

National Institutes of Health News Release. NLHBI stops trial of estrogen plus progestin due to increased breast cancer risk, lack of overall benefit (2002).

RL Prentice, et al. Conjugated equine estrogens and breast cancer risk in the Women's Health Initiative clinical trial and observational study. *American Journal of Epidemiology* 167 (2008): 1407–1415.

RL Prentice, et al. Estrogen plus progestin therapy and breast cancer in recently postmenopausal women. *American Journal of Epidemiology* 167 (2008): 1207–1216

CW Randolph and Genie James. *From Hormone Hell to Hormone Well,* Deerborn, FL: Health Communications (2009), 29.

M Ravdin, KA Cronin, N Howlander, CD Berg, RT Chlebowski, EJ Feuer, BK Edwards, and DA Berry. The decrease in breast cancer incidence in 2003 in the United States. *New England Journal of Medicine* 356(16) (2007): 1670–1674.

Tomas Riman, Paul W Dickman, Stafan Nilsson, Nestor Correia, Hans Nordlinger, Cecilia M Magnusson, Elisabete Weiderpass, and Ingermar R Persson. *Hormone Replacement Therapy and the Risk of Invasive Epithelial Ovarian Cancer in Swedish Women.* National Cancer Institute (2002).

RK Ross, A Paganini-Hill, PC Wan, and MC Pike. Effect of hormone replacement therapy on breast cancer risk. *Journal of the National Cancer Institute* 92 (2000): 328–332.

JE Rossouw, GL Anderson, RL Prentice, et al., for Writing Group for the Women's Health Initiative. Risks and benefits of estrogen plus progestin in health postmenopausal women: principal results from the Women Health Initiative. *Journal of the American Medical Association* 288 (2002): 321–333.

D Schechter. Estrogen, progesterone, and mood. *Journal of Gender-Specific Medicine* 2 (1999): 29–36.

Barbara Seaman. *The Greatest Experiment Ever Performed on Women.* New York: Hyperion (2003), 28, 212.

C Schairer, J Lubin, R Troisi, et al. Menopausal estrogen and estrogen-progestin replacement therapy and breast cancer risk. *Journal of the American Medical Association* 283 (2000): 485–494.

Sally A Shumaker, Claudine Legault, Stephen R Rapp, Leon Thal, Robert B Wallace, Judithe K Ockene, Susan L Hendrix, Beverly N Jones III, Ann-louise R Assaf, Rebecca D Jackson, Jane Morley Kotchen, Sylvia W Sassertheil-Smoller, and Jean Wactawski-Wende, for the WHIMS Investigators. Estrogen plus progestin and the incidence of dementia and mild cognitive impairment in postmenopausal women. *Journal of the American Medical Association* 291 (2003): 2947–2958.

Sally A Shumaker et al. Estrogen plus progestin and the incidence of dementia and mild cognitive impairment in postmenopausal women. *Journal of the American Medical Association* 289 (2003): 2651.

Darcy V Spicer, Giske Ursin, Yuri R Parisky, John G Pearce, Donna Shoupe, Anne Pike, and Malcolm C Pike. Changes in mammographic densities induced by a hormonal contraceptive designed to reduce breast cancer risk. *Journal of the National Cancer Institute* 86 (1994): 431–436.

L Titus-Ernstoff, EE Hatch, RN Hoover, J Palmer, ER Greenber, W Ricker, et al. Long-term cancer risk in women given diethylstilbestrol (DES) during pregnancy. *British Journal of Cancer* 84 (2001): 126–133.

MP Vessey, DVI Fairweather, B Norman-Smith, and J Buckley. A randomized double blind controlled trial of the value of diethystillbestrol therapy in pregnancy: long term follow-up of mothers and offspring. *British Journal of Obstetrics and Gynaecology* 90 (1983): 1007–1017.

MK Whiteman, Y Cui, JA Flaws, et al. Media coverage of women's health issues: is there a bias in the reporting of an association between hormone replacement therapy and breast cancer? *J Women's Health Gend Based Med.* 10 (2001): 571–577.

Duff Wilson. Publisher opens inquiry into article on Wyeth drug. *International Herald Tribune* (December 26, 2008).

Robert A Wilson. The roles of estrogen and progesterone in breast and genital cancer. *Journal of the American Medical Association* 182(327) (1962): 8.

DL Wingard and J Turiel. Long-term effects of exposure to diethylstilbestrol. *Western Journal of Medicine* 149(5) (1988): 551–554.

Women's Health Initiative Study Group. Design of the Women's Health Initiative clinical trial and observational study. *Control Clin Trials* 19 (1998): 61–109.

Jonathan V Wright and John Morgenthaler. *Natural Hormone Replacement.* Petaluma, CA: Smart Publications (1997), 23.

JV Wright. Comparative measurements of serum estriol, estradiol, and EI in non-pregnant, premenopausal women: a preliminary investigation. *Alternative Medicine Review* 4 (1999): 266–270.

Writing Group for the Women's Health Initiative. Risks and benefits of estrogen plus progestin in healthy postmenopausal women. *Journal of the American Medical Association* 288 (2002): 321–333.

Peter J Zandi, et al. Hormone replacement therapy and incidence of Alzheimer's disease in older women: the Cache County study. *Journal of the American Medical Association* 288(2123) (2002): 217–224.

Chapter 5

Lloyd V Allen, Jr. Estriol: women's choice vs. a manufacturer's greed. *International Journal of Medicine* 12(4) (2008): 289.

Marcia Angell. *The Truth About the Drug Companies—How They Deceive us and What to Do About It.* New York: Random House (2004).

T Bagis, A Gokcel, HB Zeyneloglu, E Tarim, EB Kilicdag, and B Haydardedeoglu. The effects of short-term medroxyprogesterone acetate and micronized progesterone on glucose metabolism and lipid profiles in patients with polycystic ovary syndrome: a prospective randomized study. *Journal of Clinical Endocrinology and Metabolism* 87(10) (2002): 4536–4540.

Lisa A Boothby, Paul L Doering, and Simon Kipersztok. Bioidentical hormone therapy: a review. *Menopause* 11(3) (2004): 356–367.

C Campagnoli, F Clavel-Chapelon, R Kaaks, C Peris, and F Berrino. Progestin and progesterone in hormone replacement therapy and the risk of breast cancer. *Journal of Steroid Biochemistry and Molecular Biology* 96(2) (2005): 95–108.

B De Lignieres. Effects of progestrogens on the postmenopausal breast. *Climacteric* 5(3) (2002): 229–235.

A Fournier, F Berrino, E Riboli, V Avenel, and F Clavel-Chapelon. Breast cancer risk in relation to different types of replacement therapy in the E3N-EPIC cohort. *International Journal of Cancer* 114(3) (2005): 448–454.

Deborah Grady, Bruce Ettinger, Anna Tosteson, Alice Pressman, and Judith L Macer. Predictors of difficulty when discontinuing postmenopausal hormone therapy. *Obstetrics and Gynecology* 102(6) (2003): 1233–1239.

JD Graham and CL Clarke. Physiological action of progesterone in target tissues. *Endocrine Reviews* 18(4) (1997): 502–519.

John R Lee. *Natural Progesterone—The Multiple Roles of a Remarkable Hormone.* Sebastopol, CA: BBL Publishing (1993).

John R Lee and Virginia Hopkins. *What Your Doctor May NOT Tell You About Menopause.* New York: Hachette Book Group USA (1996).

John R Lee and Virginia Hopkins. *What Your Doctor May NOT Tell You About Premenopause.* New York: Hachette Book Group USA (1999).

John R Lee, David Zava, and Virginia Hopkins. *What Your Doctor May NOT Tell You About Breast Cancer.* New York: Warner Books (2002).

HB Leonetti, J Landes, D Steinberg, and JN Anasti. Topical progesterone cream as an alternative progestin in hormone therapy. *Alternative Therapies in Health and Medicine* 11(6) (2005): 36–38.

RA Lobo. Progestogen metabolism. *Journal of Reproductive Medicine* 44(2) (1999): 148–152.

GDO Lowe. Hormone replacement therapy: prothrombotic vs. protective effects. *Pathophysiology of Haemostasis and Thrombosis* 32(5–6) (2002): 329–332.

Menopause is the beginning of a new, fulfilling stage of life, the NAMS 1997 Menopause Survey shows. *Journal of the North American Menopause Society* 5(4) (1997): 1–3

D Moskowitz. A comprehensive review of the safety and efficacy of bioidentical hormones for the management of menopause and related health risks. *Alternative Medical Review* 11(3) (2006): 208–223.

Christine Northrup. *The Wisdom of Menopause.* New York: Bantam Books (2001), 141.

D Schechter. Estrogen, progesterone, and mood. *Journal of Gender-Specific Medicine* 2 (1999): 29–36.

FZ Stanczyk. All progestins are not created equal. *Steroids* 68 (2003): 879–890.

JV Wright. Comparative measurements of serum estriol, estradiol, and E1 in nonpregnant, premenopausal women: a preliminary investigation. *Alternative Medicine Review* 4 (1999): 266–270.

Chapter 6

A Aleman, WR de Vries, EH de Haan, et al. Age-sensitive cognitive function, growth hormone and insulin-like growth factor I plasma levels in healthy older men. *Neuropsychobiology* 41(2) (2000): 73–78.

PV Carroll, ER Christ, BA Bengtsson, et al. Growth hormone deficiency in adulthood and the effects of growth hormone replacement: a review— Growth Hormone Research Society Scientific Committee. *Journal of Clinical Endocrinology and Metabolism* 83(2) (1998): 382–395.

H DeBoer, GJ Block, and EA Van der Veen. Clinical aspects of growth hormone deficiency in adults. *Endocrine Review* 1 (1995): 63–86.

R Fernholm, M Bramnert, E Hagg, et al. Growth hormone replacement therapy improves body composition and increases bone metabolism in elderly patients with pituitary disease. *Journal of Clinical Endocrinology and Metabolism* 85(11)(2000): 4104–4112.

C Lauritzen. Results of a 5 year prospective study of estriol succinate treatment in patients with climacteric complaints. *Hormone and Metabolic Research* 19(11)(1987): 579–584.

M Melamed, E Castano, AC Notides, and S Sasson. Molecular and kinetic basis for the mixed agonist/antagonist activity of estriol. *Molecular Endocrinology* 11(12)(1997): 868–878.

AM Olivia, ND Franks, and Jonathan V Wright. Estriol: its weakness is its strength. *Life Extension Magazine* (August 21–24, 2008).

A Sartorio, A Conti, E Molinari, et al. Growth hormone and cognitive functions. *Hormone Research* 45(1–2)(1996): 23–29.

K Takahasi, M Okada, T Ozaki, et al. Safety and efficacy of oestriol for symptoms of natural or surgically induced menopause. *Hormone Research* 15(5)(2000): 1028–1036.

AA Toogood and SM Shalet. Ageing and growth hormone status. *Baillieres Clinical Endocrinology Metabolism* 12(2)(1998): 281–296.

VA Tzingounis, MF Aksu, and RB Greenblatt. Estriol in management of the menopause. *Journal of the American Medical Association* 239(16)(1978): 1638–1641.

PS van Dam, A Aleman, WR de Vries, et al. Growth hormone, insulin-like growth factor I and cognitive function in adults. *Growth Horm IGF Res* 10(suppl. B)(2000): S69–S73.

TS Yang, SH Tsan, SP Chang, and HT Ng. Efficacy and safety of estriol replacement therapy for climacteric women. *Zhonghua Yi Xue Za Zhi* (Taipei) 55(5)(1995): 386–391.

Chapters 7 and 8

P Albertazzi, F Pansini, G Bonaccorsi, L Zanotti, E Forini, and D DeAloysio. The effect of dietary soy supplementation on hot flushes. *Obstetrics and Gynecology* 91 (1998): 6–11.

Antioxidants rock: inside your body, an army of antioxidants is protecting you from the forces of aging and disease. We're huge fans of these stellar nutrients and how you can get more on your side. *Women's Health Magazine* (December 3, 2007), 1–3.

J Bowe, XF Li, J Kinsey-Jones, et al. The hop phytoestrogen, 8-prenylnaringenin, reverses the ovariectomy-induced rise in skin temperatures in an animal model of menopausal hot flushes. *Journal of Endocrinology* 191(2) (2006): 399–405.

F Branca and S Lorenzetti. Health effects of phytoestrogen. *Form Nutr* 57 (2005): 100–11.

T Cornwell, W Cohick, and I Raskin. Dietary phytoestrogens and health. *Phytochemistry* 65(8) (2004): 995–1006.

M Cosentino, F Marino, M Ferrari, et al. Estrogenic activity of 7-hydroxymatairesinol potassium acetate (HMR/lignan) from Norway spruce *(Picea abies)* knots and of its active metabolite enterolactone in MCF-7 cells. *Pharmacological Research* 56(2) (2007): 140–147.

D De Keukeleire CL De, H Rong, et al. Functional properties of hop polyphenols. *Basic Life Science* 66 (1999): 739–760.

D De Keukeleire, L De Cooman, H Rong, A Heyerick, J Kalita, and SR Milligan. Functional properties of hop polyphenols. *Basic Life Science* 66 (1999): 739–760.

MJ de Kleign, YT van der Schouw, PW Wilson, DE Grobbee, and PF Jacques. Dietary intake of phytoestrogens is associated with a favorable metabolic cardiovascular risk profile in postmenopausal US women: the Framingham study. *Journal of Nutrition* 132(2) (2002): 276–282.

Dietary Guidelines for Americans (2005), Office of Disease Prevention and Health Promotion, U.S. Department of Health and Human Services, www.health.gov/dietaryguidelines/dga.2005/document.

SE File, N Jarrett, E Fluck, et al. Eating soya improves human memory. *Psychopharmacology* (Berlin) 157(4) (2001): 430–436.

JH Fowke, C Longcope, and JR Herbert. Brassica vegetable consumption shifts estrogen metabolism in healthy postmenopausal women. *Cancer Epidemiology Biomarkers and Prevention* 9(8) (2000): 773–779.

OH Franco, H Burger, CE Lebrun, et al. Higher dietary intake of lignans is associated with better cognitive performance in postmenopausal women. *Journal of Nutrition* 135(5) (2005): 1190–1195.

SE Fugate and CO Church. Nonestrogen treatment modalities for vasomotor symptoms associated with menopause. *Annals of Pharmacotherapy* 38(9) (2004): 1482–1499.

Renu Gandhi and Suzanne M. Snedeker. Consumer concerns about hormones in food. Cornell University, Fact Sheet No. 37 (June 2000), www.envirocancer.cornell.edu/Factsheet/Diet/fs37.hormones.cfm.

SE Geller and L Studee. Botanical and dietary supplements for menopausal symptoms: what works, what does not. *Journal of Women's Health* (Larchmont) 14(7) (2005): 634–649.

CJ Haggans, AM Hutchins, BA Olson, W Thomas, MC Martini, and JL Slavin. Effect of flaxseed consumption on urinary estrogen metabolites in postmenopausal women. *Nutrition and Cancer* 33(2) (1999): 188–195.

KK Han, JM Soares, MA Haidar, G Rodrigues de Lima, and EC Baracat. Benefits of soy isoflavone therapeutic regimen on menopausal symptoms. *Obstetrics and Gynecology* 99 (2002): 389–394.

M Hedelin, A Klint, ET Chang, et al. Dietary phytoestrogen, serum enterolactone and risk of prostate cancer: the cancer prostate Sweden study. *Cancer Causes Control* 17(2) (2006): 169–180.

A Heyerick, S Vervarcke, H Depypere, M Bracke, and KD De. A first prospective, randomized, double-blind placebo-controlled study on the use of a standardized hop extract to alleviate menopausal discomforts. *Maturitas* 54(2) (2006): 164–175.

JD Hirata, LM Swiersz, B Zell, R Small, and B Ettinger. Does dong quai have estrogenic effects in postmenopausal women? A double-blind, placebo-controlled trial. *Fertility and Sterility* 68(6) (1997): 981–986.

M Jenab and LU Thompson. The influence of flaxseed and lignans on colon carcinogenesis and beta-glucuronidase activity. *Carcinogensis* 17(6) (1996): 1343–1348.

L Kangas, N Saarinen, M Mutanen, et al. Antioxidant and antitumor effects of hydroxymatairesinol (HM-3000, HMR), a lignan isolated from the knots of spruce. *European Journal of Cancer Prevention* 114(2) (2002): S48–S57.

Dale Kiefer. A natural approach to menopause. *Life Extension Magazine* (April 2006), 3–6.

MK Kim, BC Chung, VY Yu, et al. Relationships of urinary phyto-oestrogen excretion to BMD in postmenopausal women. *Clinical Endocrinology* (Oxford) 56(3) (2002): 321–328.

S Kreijkamp-Kaspers, L Kok, ML Bots, DE Grobbee, YT van der Schouw. Dietary phytoestrogens and vascular function in postmenopausal women: a cross-sectional study. *Journal of Hypertension* 22(7) (2004): 1381–1388.

Mindy S Kurzer. Phytoestrogen supplement use by women. *Journal of Nutrition* 133 (2003): 1983S–1986S.

MS Kurzer and X Xu. Dietary phytoestrogens. *Annual Review of Nutrition* 17 (1997): 353–381.

James B LaValle and Ernest Hawkins. Nutritional support for the menopausal patient. *OB/GYN Special Edition* (2000): 55–57.

Lane Lenard. Relieving menopausal symptoms naturally. *Life Extension Magazine* (February 2009), 31–36.

AE Lethaby, J Brown, J Marjoribanks, F Kronenberg, H Roberts, and J Eden. Phytoestrogens for vasomotor menopausal symptoms. *Cochrane Database System Review* 17(4) (2007): CD001395.

J Linseisen, R Piller, S Hermann, and J Chang-Claude. Dietary phytoestrogen intake and premenopausal breast cancer risk in a German case-control study. *International Journal of Cancer* 110(2) (2004): 284–290.

LW Lissin and JP Cooke. Phytoestrogens and cardiovascular health. *Journal of the American College of Cardiology* 35(6) (2000): 1403–1410.

G Livera, et al. Regulation and perturbation of testicular functions by vitamin A. *Reproduction* 124 (2002): 173–180.

C Longcope, HA Feldman, JB Mc Kinlay, and AB Araujo. Diet and sex hormone-binding globulin. *Journal of Clinical Endocrinology and Metabolism* 85(1) (2000): 293–296.

R Lupu, I Mehmi, E Atlas, et al. Black cohosh, a menopausal remedy, does not have estrogenic activity and does not promote breast cancer cell growth. *International Journal of Oncology* 23(5) (2003): 1407–1412.

GB Mahady. Black cohosh (*Actgaea/Cimicifuga racemosa*): review of the clinical data for safety and efficacy in menopausal symptoms. *Treat Endocrinol* 4(3) (2005): 177–184.

Mayo Clinic Staff. Cholesterol: the top 5 foods to lower your numbers. MayoClinic.com (2008).

SE McCann, P Muti, D Vito, et al. Dietary lignan intakes and risk of pre- and postmenopausal breast cancer. *International Journal of Cancer* 111(3) (2004): 440–443.

DM Minich and JS Bland. A review of the clinical efficacy and safety of cruciferous vegetable phytochemicals. *Nutrition Review* 65(65, pt. 1) (2007): 259–267.

C Nagata, S Inaba, N Kawakami, T Kakizoe, and H Shimizu. Inverse association of soy product intake with serum androgen and estrogen concentrations in Japanese men. *Nutrition Cancer* 36(1) (2000): 14–18.

C Nagata, N Takatsuka, N Kawakami, and H Shimizu. Soy product intake and hot flashes in Japanese women: results from a community-based prospective study. *American Journal of Epidemiology* 153 (2001): 790–793.

Natural ways to combat testosterone loss. *Life Extension Magazine* (February 24, 2004).

Aurora M Nedelcu and Richard E Michod. Sex as a response to oxidative stress: the effect of antioxidants on sexual induction in a facultatively sexual lineage. *Royal Society* 270 (2003): S136–S139.

A Netter, R Hartoma, and K Nahoul. Effect of zinc administration on plasma testosterone, dihydrotestosterone and sperm count. *Artch Androl* 7(1)(1981): 69–73.

R Osmer, M Friede, E Liske, et al. Efficacy and safety of isopropanolic black cohosh extract for climacteric symptoms. *Obstetrics and Gynecology* 105(5, pt. I)(2005): 1074–1083.

BA Pockaj, CL Loprinzi, JA Sloan, et al. Pilot evaluation of black cohosh for the treatment of hot flashes in women. *Cancer Investigation* 22(4)(2004): 515–521.

B Roemheld-Hamm. Chasteberry. *American Family Physician* 72(5)(2005): 821–824.

NM Saarinen, PE Penttinen, AL Smeds, TT Hurmerinta, and SI Makela. Structural determinants of plant lignans for growth of mammary tumors and hormonal responses in vivo. *Journal of Steroid Biochemistry and Molecular Biology* 93(2–5)(2005): 209–219.

M Saleem, HJ Kim, MS Ali, and YS Lee. An update on bioactive plant lignans. *Natural Products Report* 22(6)(2005): 696–716.

MB Schabath, LM Hernandez, X Wu, PC Pillow, and MR Spitz. Dietary phytoestrogens and lung cancer risk. *Journal of the American Medical Association* 294(12)(2005): 1493–1504.

NP Seeram, LS Adams, SM Henning, et al. In vitro antiproliferative, apoptotic and antioxidant activities of punicalagin, ellagic acid and a total pomegranate tannin extract are enhanced in combination with other polyphenols as found in pomegranate juice. *Journal of Nutritional Biochemistry* 16(6)(2005): 360–367.

S Sehmisch, F Hammer, J Christoffel, et al. Comparison of the phytohormones genistein, resveratrol and 8-prenylnaringenin as agents for preventing osteoporosis. *Planta Medical* 74(8)(2008): 794–801.

D Seidlove-Wuttke, O Hesse, H Jarry, et al. Evidence for selective estrogen receptor modulator activity in a black cohosh *(Cimicifuga racemosa)* extract: comparison with estradiol-17 beta. *European Journal of Endocrinology* 149(4)(2003): 351–362.

M Serraino and LU Thompson. Flaxseed supplementation and early markers of colon carcinogenesis. *Cancer Letter* 63(2) (1992): 15–65.

MK Sung, M Lautens, and LU Thompson. Mammalian lignans inhibit the growth of estrogen-independent human colon tumor cells. *Anticancer Research* 18(3A) (1998): 1405–1408.

H Takihara, MJ Cosentino, and AT Cockett. Zinc sulfate therapy for infertile males with or without varicocelectomy. *Urology* 29(6) (1987): 638–641.

M Tikkiwal, RL Ajmera, and NK Mathur. Effect of zinc administration on seminal zinc and fertility of oligospermic males. *Indian Journal of Physiology and Pharmacology* 31(1) (1987): 30–34.

S Turner and S Mills. A double-blind clinical trial on herbal remedy for premenstrual syndrome: a case study. *Complementary Therapies in Medicine* 1 (1993): 73–77.

DH Upmalis, R Lobo, L Bradley M Warren, FL Cone, and CA Lamia. Vasomotor symptom relief by soy isoflavone extract tablets in postmenopausal women: a multicenter, double-blind, randomized, placebo-controlled study. *Menopause* 7 (2000): 236–242.

S Washburn, GL Burke, T Morgan, and M Anthony. Effect of soy protein supplementation on serum lipoproteins, blood pressure and menopausal women. *Menopause* 6 (1999): 7–13.

W Wuttke, H Jarry, V Christoffel, B Spengler, and D Seidlova-Wuttke. Chaste tree *(Vitex agnus-castus)*—pharmacology and clinical indications. *Phytomedicine* 10(4) (2003): 348–357.

WH Xu, W Zheng, YB Xiang, et al. Soya food intake and risk of endometrial cancer among Chinese women in Shanghai population based case control study. *British Medical Journal* 328(7451) (2004): 1285.

X Zhang, XO Shu, H Li, et al. Prospective cohort study of soy food consumption and risk of bone fracture among postmenopausal women. *Archives of Internal Medicine* 165(16) (2005): 1890–1895.

Chapter 9

A Bylund, N Saarinen, JX Zhang, et al. Anticancer effects of a plant lignan 7-hydroxymatairesinol on a prostate cancer model in vivo. *Experimental Biology and Medicine* (Maywood) 230(3) (2005): 217–223.

MP Carey and BT Johnson. Effectiveness of yohimbine in the treatment of erectile disorder: four eta-analytic integrations. *Archives of Sexual Behavior* 25 (1996): 341.

G Cavallini, S Caracciolo, G Vitali, et al. Carnitine versus androgen administration in the treatment of sexual dysfunction, depressed mood, and fatigue associated with male aging. *Urology* 63 (2004): 641–646.

J Chen, Y Wollman, T Chernichovsky, et al. Effect of oral administration of high-dose nitric oxide donor L-arginine in men with organic erectile dysfunction: results of a double-blind, randomized study. *British Journal of Urology International* 83 (1999): 269–273.

W Cherdshewasart and N Nimsakul. Clinical trial of *Butea superba*, an alternative herbal treatment for erectile dysfunction. *Asian Journal of Andrology* 5 (2003): 243–246.

HK Choi, DH Seong, and KH Rha. Clinical efficacy of Korean red ginseng for erectile dysfunction. *International Journal of Impotence Research* 7 (1995): 181–186.

AJ Cohen and B Bartlik. Ginkgo biloba for antidepressant-induced sexual dysfunction. *Journal of Sex and Marital Therapy* 24 (1989): 139–143.

GF Combs and WP Gray. Chemopreventive agents: selenium. *Pharmacology and Theraputics* 79(3) (1998): 179–192.

M Condra, A Moralex, JA Owen, et al. Prevalence and significance of tobacco smoking in impotence. *Urology* 27 (1986): 495–498.

Z Durackova, B Trebaticky, V Novotny, et al. Lipid metabolism and erectile function improvement by Pycnogenol, extract from the bark of *Pinus pinaster*, in patients suffering from erectile dysfunction—a pilot study. *Nutrition Research* 23 (2003): 1189–1198.

E Ernst and MH Pittler. Yohimbine for erectile dysfunction: a systematic review and meta-analysis of randomized clinical trials. *Journal of Urology* 159 (1998): 433–436.

K Esposito, F Giugliano, C Di Palo, et al. Effect of lifestyle changes on erectile dysfunction in obese men: a randomized controlled trial. *Journal of the American Medical Association* 291 (2004): 2978–2984.

E Giovannucci, et al. Study of prediagnostic selenium levels in toenails and the risk of advanced prostate cancer. *Journal of the National Cancer Institute* 90(16) (1998): 1219–1224.

MD Hendler and Saul Sheldon. *The Doctor's Vitamin and Mineral Encyclopedia.* New York: Fireside (1990), 209–215.

C Hernandez-Lopez. Drugs do not only relieve male menopause. *British Medical Journal* (2000): 321–451.

B Hong, YH Ji, JH Hong, et al. A double-blind crossover study evaluating the efficacy of Korean red ginseng in patients with erectile dysfunction: a preliminary report. *Journal of Urology* 168 (2002): 2070–2073.

TY Ito, AS Trant, and ML Polan. A double-blind placebo-controlled study of ArginMax, a nutritional supplement for enhancement of female sexual function. *Journal of Sex and Marital Therapy* 27(5) (2001): 541–549.

T Klotz, MJ Mathers, M Braun, W Bloch, and U Engelmann. Effectiveness of oral L-arginine in first-line treatment of erectile dysfunction in a controlled crossover study. *Urology International* 63(4) (1999): 220–223.

L Konrad, HH Muller, C Lenz, H Laubinger, G Aumuller, and JJ Lichius. Antiproliferative effect on human prostate cancer cells by a stinging nettle root *(Urtica dioica)* extract. *Planta Medical* 66(1) (2000): 44–47.

P Kunelius, J Hakkinen, and O Lukkarinen. Is high-dose yohimbine hydrochloride effective in the treatment of mixed-type impotence? A prospective, randomized, controlled double-blind crossover study. *Urology* 49 (1997): 441–444

NA Lopatikin, et al. Combined extract of Sabal palm and nettle in the treatment of patients with lower urinary tract symptoms in double blind, placebo-controlled trial. *Urologiia* 12(2) (2006): 14–19.

K Mann, T Klinger, S Noe, et al. Effect of yohimbine on sexual experiences and nocturnal tumescence and rigidity in erectile dysfunction. *Archives of Sexual Behavior* 25 (1996): 1–16.

D McKay. Nutrients and botanicals for erectile dysfunction: examining the evidence. *Alternative Medicine Review* 1 (2004): 4–16.

EA Melo, et al. Evaluating the efficiency of a combination of *Pygeum africanum* and stinging nettle *(Urtica dioica)* extracts in treating benign prostatic hyperplasia (BPH): double-blind, randomized, placebo controlled trial. *International Brazilian Journal of Urology* 28(5) (2002): 418–425.

CM Meston and M Worcel. The effects of yohimbine plus L-arginine glutamate on sexual arousal in postmenopausal women with sexual arousal disorder. *Archives of Sexual Behavior* 31(4) (2002): 323–332.

JA Moody, D Vernet, S Laidlaw, J Rajfer, and NF Gonzalez-Cadavid. Effects of long-term oral administration of L-arginine on the rat erectile response. *Journal of Urology* 158(3 pt. 1) (1997): 942–947.

G Popa, et al. Efficacy of a combined *Sabal-urtica* preparation in the symptomatic treatment of benign prostatic hyperplasia. Results of a placebo-controlled double-blind study. *MMW Fortschritte der Medizin* 147(3) (2005): 103–108.

WJ Reiter, A Pycha, G Schatzi, et al. Dehydroepiandrosterone in the treatment of erectile dysfunction: a prospective, double-blind randomized, placebo-controlled study. *Urology* 53 (1999): 590–595.

Ray Sahelian. Dietary supplementation with L-arginine or placebo in women with preeclampsia. Staff AC. Departments of Obstetrics and Gynecology. *Ulleval University Hospital, Kirkeveien,* Oslo, Norway (1995).

Ray Sahelian. Treatment of erectile dysfunction with pycnogenol and L-arginine. *Journal of Sex and Marital Therapy* 29(3) (2003): 207–213.

Ray Sahelian. The influence of two different doses of L-arginine oral supplementation on nitric oxide (NO) concentration and total antioxidants status (TAS) in atherosclerotic patients. *Medical Science Monitor* 10(1) (2004): CR29–C32.

Christopher S Saigal. Obesity and erectile dysfunction, common problems, common solutions? *Journal of the American Medical Association* 291(24) (2004): 3011–3012.

M Sohn and R Sikora. Ginkgo biloba extract in the therapy of erectile dysfunction. *Journal of Sex Education and Therapy* 17 (1991): 53–61.

C Walther, et al. Benign prostatic syndrome. Urinary urgency and micturition frequency reduced with plant preparation. *MMW Fortschr. Med.* 147(40) (2005): 52–53.

AW Zorgniotti and EF Lizza. Effect of large doses of the nitric oxide precursor, L-arginine, on erectile dysfunction. *International Journal of Impotence Research* 6 (1994): 33–36.

Chapter 11

Klein L Cousino and EJ Corwin. Seeing the unexpected: how sex differences in stress responses may provide a new perspective on the manifestation of psychiatric disorders. *Current Psychiatry Reports* 4(6) (2002): 441–448.

Grant P Cumming, Heather D Currie, Rik Moncur, and Amanda J Lee. Web-based survey on the effect of menopause on women's libido in a computer-literate population. *Royal Society of Medicine Press Limited Menopause International* 15(1) (2009): 8–12.

R Doll. One for the heart. *British Medical Journal* 315 (1997): 164–168.

DC Geary and MV Flinn. Sex differences in behavioral and hormonal response to social threat: commentary on Taylor et al. *Psychological Review* 109(4) (2002): 745–750; discussion 751–753.

M Leitzmann, et al. Frequency of ejaculation and risk of prostate cancer. *Journal of the American Medical Association* 292 (2004): 329.

S Gottlieb. Frequent ejaculation may be linked to decreased risk of prostate cancer. *British Medical Journal* 328 (2004): 851.

W James. A hypothesis on the sexual behavior of men who are destined to develop prostate cancer. *International Journal of Epidemology* 34 (2005): 483–485.

Lindau, et al. Sexuality and health among older adults in the United States. *New England Journal of Medicine* 357 (2007): 2732–2733.

Chapter 12

Tanya E Davison and Marita P McCabe. Relationships between men's and women's body image and their psychological, social, and sexual functioning. *Sex Roles: A Journal of Research* (52 7–8) April 2005, 463–475 (13).

Richard Nicastro. How to deepen intimacy through the power of empathic listening. www.articlebase.com (2008).

Marianne Williamson. *The Age of Miracles.* California: Hay House (2008), xvii.

ACKNOWLEDGMENTS

This book is a personal and professional testimony brought to life through the stories of many individuals. We extend our deepest gratitude to the patients who encouraged and nudged us to create a larger platform for sharing our science-based, natural formula for great sex, hormone balance, and better health at every age. We are also greatly indebted to many gifted individuals who inspired, guided, and contributed to this book.

First and foremost, a very big thank you to our agent, Jill Marsal, for her willingness to listen to a cold-call pitch and then work with us to pull out all the stops to make this book happen. Jill's razor-sharp candor coupled with her astute mediating skills proved to be our most trusted ally.

This book would never have become a reality without the enthusiasm, talent, and input of our publishing team at Simon & Schuster. Most especially, we express deep thanks to our outstanding editor, Michelle Howry, for believing in the merit of this project and sharing with us her editing wisdom, consistent encouragement, and special sparkle of wit. Also, we are especially grateful to Marcia Burch and Kelly Bowen for their ready willingness to champion this book while deftly guiding us through the moray of book marketing and public relations activities.

Our combined expertise and perspective on natural approaches for boosting lagging hormone levels to restore libido and sexual performance have developed over decades. We are extremely fortunate to have shared ideas and outcomes with many brilliant minds who, in turn, have encouraged, challenged, and inspired us to take a stand on a national front. First and foremost, we want to acknowledge the late John R. Lee, M.D., medical pioneer in the field of bioidentical hormone replacement and primary author of *What Your Doctor May NOT Tell You About Premenopause, What Your Doctor May NOT Tell You About Menopause,* and *What Your Doctor May NOT Tell You About Breast Cancer.* We also want to thank Joel Hargrove, M.D., for his willingness to oppose the pharmaceutical industry via his tenacity for groundbreaking medical research in the field of bioidentical hormone replacement; Christiane Northrup, M.D., for her unmistakable voice and published works that first helped introduce the term *bioidentical* into the layperson's vocabulary; Erika Schwartz, M.D., for her strength and courage as a spokeswoman for our cause; Helene Leonetti, M.D., for her research substantiating the clinical benefits of bioidentical progesterone replacement; Joann E. Manson, M.D., for her work in preventive medicine and hormone replacement; Kenna Stephenson, M.D., for her research examining how bioidentical hormone replacement positively influences women's cardiovascular health and aging process; James L. Wilson, M.D., for his illuminating work on the adrenal hormones; and David

Zava, Ph.D., for his daring research linking breast cancer and synthetic hormone replacement. We want to acknowledge Virginia Hopkins for her pivotal role in working with Dr. Lee to coauthor the above-mentioned three books that set the stage for the current revolution supporting the use of bioidentical hormone therapies, and to thank Candace Burch for her persistent and eloquent efforts to educate the consumer about safe and efficacious choices for hormone balancing. Also, special kudos to Sharon McFarland, Jane Murray, M.D., and Deb Soholt, R.N., for founding Women in Balance, a national, nonprofit organization dedicated to empowering women to take charge of their hormone health.

In this era, when pharmaceutical marketing risks skew medical research data, we applaud the leadership teams at both the Professional Compounding Center of America (PCCA) and the International Association of Compounding Pharmacies (IACP) for their stamina in fighting the money-for-power exchange that goes on between pharmaceutical lobbyists and members of Congress. We are also excited by the strides that these two organizations, as well as Jim Paoletti at ZRT Laboratory, are making in educating the medical community regarding the safety and efficacy of bioidentical hormone replacement.

We are also delighted to celebrate the cacophony of celebrity voices that are helping bioidentical hormone replacement therapy (BHRT) become a household term. In 2009, women who had not been able to establish a meaningful dialogue with their physicians about menopausal symptoms and hormone health concerns tuned into television specials hosted by Oprah and Robin McGraw to learn about BHRT. Within the hour that each program aired, our medical practice was swamped with hundreds of phone calls from women wanting an individualized hormone health consultation. Across the nation, the ripple effect soon became a tidal wave forcing the traditional medical community to get its collective heads out of the sand and take notice of the science supporting the safety and efficacy of BHRT.

Books do not pop out of a computer printer fully formed. This book would never have moved from concept to reality without the tenacious support of many individuals on our home front. Special thanks to our superlative team at the Dalton Agency, specifically Michael Munz, Jim Dalton, Melissa Ross, and Brendan Cumiskey, for helping to position us as accessible and solid resources for reliable information on hormone health issues. A heartfelt thanks also to Nannette Noffsinger, media and public relations consultant, for her ever-present faith and humor combined with an unsurpassed ability to weave a network of contacts into a tapestry of events and media happenings.

Many thanks to Jennifer Hobbs, marketing coordinator and patient liaison for the Natural Hormone Institute. This book would never have been completed without Jennifer's tireless willingness to bounce multiple balls with very little guidance. Also, we thank our office staff—most particularly Michelle Rossi, Susan Shee, Sherri Kitchens, and Michelle Neely—for managing the day-to-day environment where healing hormone health actually occurs.

We also want to acknowledge our Ageless and Wellness Center's staff of medical professionals: Patti Landry, A.R.N.P., Nicole Aldrich, A.R.N.P., Anna Stauch, A.R.N.P., and Lisa Lynch, P.A. Treating women and men with hormone health issues can be challenging, but our medical professionals blend their unique medical expertise with compassion, pragmatism, and a holistic approach to treatment and care. It is because of the skills and commitment of these women that our medical practice is able to serve patients from far and wide.

Finally, our deepest gratitude extends to our patients. Thank you for entrusting us to discuss and address your sexual health concerns. Even more, thank you for informing and teaching us through your stories. It is our hope that this book will allow your voice to contribute to the crescendo demanding hormone health—and a rewarding sex life—at every age.

INDEX

ABOUT THE AUTHORS

Genie James, M.M.Sc., is the chief executive officer of the Ageless and Wellness Medical Center and cofounder of the Natural Hormone Institute with Dr. C. W. Randolph, Jr. She has been nationally recognized by the Healthcare Financial Management Association, the National Association of Women's Health, and the University of California's Center for Health Professions as a powerful change-agent in the areas of consumer-driven health care and natural, or integrative, medicine. In 2007, she founded Women Evolving, LLC, an organization dedicated to educating women about how they can use their choice, voice, and financial power to enhance their personal health care while positively impacting our nation's overall health care delivery system. Ms. James is the coauthor of *From Hormone Hell to Hormone Well* and *From Belly Fat to Belly Flat* with Dr. Randolph. For more information, go to www.hormonewell.com.

C. W. Randolph, Jr., M.D., one of the nation's leading bioidentical hormone physician-experts, has treated thousands of women and men with hormone imbalances for more than a decade. A graduate of Louisiana State University School of Medicine, Dr. Randolph is board certified by the American College of Obstetrics and Gynecology as well as the American Board of Holistic Medicine. He is also board certified by the International Academy of Compounding Pharmacists and is on the faculty for national physicians continuing medical education (CME) programs hosted by the Professional Compounding Centers of America, ZRT Laboratory, and College Pharmacy. Dr Randolph's Ageless and Wellness Medical Center (www.agelessandwellness.com) treats more than eight thousand patients each year. As the cofounder of the Natural Hormone Institute (NHI), Dr. Randolph interfaces with women and men across the globe via www.hormonewell.com.